Compassionate Person-Centered Care for the Dying

7/16

Bonnie Freeman, DNP, ANP, RN, ACHPN, is an adult nurse practitioner in the Department of Supportive Care Medicine at the City of Hope National Medical Center in Duarte, California. She is involved with treating the symptom management needs of many chronically and terminally ill individuals diagnosed with various forms of cancer. Dr. Freeman trained at such excellent facilities as the in-patient units at San Diego Hospice and the Institute of Palliative Medicine in San Diego, California, and the home care hospice program in Owensboro, Kentucky. While in Kentucky, she completed her advanced practice clinical training for adult nurse practitioners with a specialty focus on palliative care through Vanderbilt University in Nashville, Tennessee. This program exposed Dr. Freeman to current concepts in caring for the dying, and enhanced her already significant clinical experience caring for dying individuals acquired from over 30 years working in critical care. Dr. Freeman obtained her MSN from Indiana Wesleyan University, and her DNP from Azusa Pacific University in Azusa, California.

Contributors

Tracey Das Gupta, MN, RN, CON, is director of Interprofessional Practice at Sunnybrook Health Sciences Centre in Toronto, Ontario, Canada. She is also the colead of the Quality Dying Initiative with Dr. Jeff Myers. Tracey has been passionate about health care, quality of life, and leadership since becoming a nurse in 1991. Her decision to become a nurse was influenced by her father who lived with muscular dystrophy. Ms. Das Gupta has fulfilled various frontline nursing roles along the continuum of care and has had the opportunity to continue to grow in leadership roles such as educator, professional practice leader, and director of nursing practice. In her current role, she also provides leadership for the development and implementation of Sunnybrook's interprofessional care (IPC) strategy.

Margaret Fitch, PhD, MScN, is a nurse researcher and holds an appointment at the Bloomberg Faculty of Nursing and School of Graduate Studies at the University of Toronto. She also serves as expert lead for cancer survivorship and patient experience for the Person-Centered Perspective Portfolio of the Canadian Partnership Against Cancer. She is also editor-in-chief for the *Canadian Oncology Nursing Journal*. Dr. Fitch has an extensive publication record based on her many years of research regarding patient perspectives, coping and adaptation with illness, and screening for psychosocial distress. She has particular expertise in measurement and evaluation, qualitative methods, and knowledge integration. During her career, she has held clinical and administrative positions and has maintained an ongoing role in education of both undergraduate and graduate students and health professionals in practice.

Compassionate Person-Centered Care for the Dying

An Evidence-Based
Palliative Care Guide
for Nurses

Bonnie Freeman, DNP, ANP, RN, ACHPN

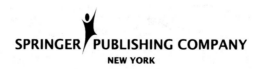

SPRINGER PUBLISHING COMPANY
NEW YORK

Copyright © 2015 Springer Publishing Company, LLC

All rights reserved.

No part of this publication may be reproduced, stored in a retrieval system, or transmitted in any form or by any means, electronic, mechanical, photocopying, recording, or otherwise, without the prior permission of Springer Publishing Company, LLC, or authorization through payment of the appropriate fees to the Copyright Clearance Center, Inc., 222 Rosewood Drive, Danvers, MA 01923, 978-750-8400, fax 978-646-8600, info@copyright.com or on the Web at www.copyright.com.

Springer Publishing Company, LLC
11 West 42nd Street
New York, NY 10036
www.springerpub.com

Acquisitions Editor: Elizabeth Nieginski
Composition: Cenveo Publisher Services

ISBN: 978-0-8261-2247-6
e-book ISBN: 978-0-8261-2248-3
CARES tool ISBN: 978-0-8261-2822-5

Student Supplements are available from http://www.springerpub.com/compassionate-person-supplemental-materials

16 17 18/5 4 3 2

The author and the publisher of this work have made every effort to use sources believed to be reliable to provide information that is accurate and compatible with the standards generally accepted at the time of publication. Because medical science is continually advancing, our knowledge base continues to expand. Therefore, as new information becomes available, changes in procedures become necessary. We recommend that the reader always consult current research and specific institutional policies before performing any clinical procedure. The author and publisher shall not be liable for any special, consequential, or exemplary damages resulting, in whole or in part, from the readers' use of, or reliance on, the information contained in this book. The publisher has no responsibility for the persistence or accuracy of URLs for external or third-party Internet websites referred to in this publication and does not guarantee that any content on such websites is, or will remain, accurate or appropriate.

Library of Congress Cataloging-in-Publication Data

Freeman, Bonnie (Bonnie J.), author.
  Compassionate person-centered care for the dying : an evidence-based palliative care guide for nurses / Bonnie Freeman.
    p. ; cm.
  Includes bibliographical references and index.
  ISBN 978-0-8261-2247-6 (alk. paper) — ISBN 978-0-8261-2248-3 (e-book) — ISBN (invalid) 978-0-8261-2822-5 (CARES tool)
  I. Title.
  [DNLM: 1. Hospice and Palliative Care Nursing. 2. Evidence-Based Nursing—methods. 3. Palliative Care—methods. 4. Patient-Centered Care. 5. Terminal Care—methods. WY 152.3]
  R726.8
  616.02'9—dc23

                                                                    2014047744

Special discounts on bulk quantities of our books are available to corporations, professional associations, pharmaceutical companies, health care organizations, and other qualifying groups. If you are interested in a custom book, including chapters from more than one of our titles, we can provide that service as well.

For details, please contact:
Special Sales Department, Springer Publishing Company, LLC
11 West 42nd Street, 15th Floor, New York, NY 10036-8002
Phone: 877-687-7476 or 212-431-4370; Fax: 212-941-7842
E-mail: sales@springerpub.com

Printed in the United States of America by Gasch Printing.

I would like to dedicate this book to Dr. Chatchada Karanes for her inspiration and trust in me; Betty Ferrell, for her support and faith in me; my husband Allen, for his understanding and love; my daughter Anna, for always being there for me; the administrators of the Departments of Nursing and Supportive Care Medicine at the City of Hope; and the faculty at Azusa Pacific University, for their never-ending faith and encouragement in promoting the use of the CARES tool.

Contents

PART IV: BARRIERS AND CHALLENGES

PART V: ADDITIONAL APPLICATIONS

PART VI: LEADING CHANGE—STORIES AND PERSPECTIVES FROM SUNNYBROOK

PART VII: CONCLUSIONS AND RESOURCES

Foreword

Caring for people in the final hours of their lives is one of the most important and sacred aspects of nursing practice. This care at the end of life is truly whole-person care, attending to physical, psychological, social, and spiritual well-being. It is also what Florence Nightingale noted as the art of nursing.

This book on CARES is a valuable contribution to the evolving field of palliative nursing care. It is authored by a model for this field, Bonnie Freeman, DNP, ANP, RN, ACHPN, and brings to the bedside what her Practice embodies—evidence-based clinically expert care. I had the privilege of serving on Bonnie's capstone committee for her Doctor of Nursing Practice degree as well as observing her in practice at the City of Hope Medical Center. Importantly, the CARES tool is far more than a product of her doctoral studies. It is the product of decades of nursing practice and her deep compassion for patients and families. It is wonderful to see brilliant nurses find each other across countries, and thus the collaboration of Bonnie with Margaret Fitch, PhD, MScN, and Tracey Das Gupta, MN, RN, CON, has now given birth to this excellent book.

A very important aspect of the CARES tool is that it acknowledges both the profound privilege we have in caring for patients at the end of life and also the compassion fatigue of nurses as a result of this work.

The CARES tool is a long-needed resource and we are all grateful to the author for moving her passion to paper. It will touch the lives and deaths of patients, families, and the nurses who care for them.

Betty Ferrell, PhD, RN, MA, FAAN, FCPN, CHPN
Professor and Director
Division of Nursing Research and Education
City of Hope
National Medical Center
Duarte, California

Preface

The CARES tool was designed to be an acronym-organized and condensed education reference that provides prompts and recommendations to consider when caring for the dying. It is based on five common symptom management needs typically addressed when caring for the dying, identified from a literature review and analysis. The CARES tool was introduced to health care providers through poster presentations at national conferences in 2012, and in an article titled "CARES: An Acronym Organized Tool for the Care of the Dying," published in the *Journal of Hospice and Palliative Nursing* in May 2013.

The CARES tool article was the most downloaded article on MedScape in May 2013. Response to the CARES tool continues to be very positive, and I continue to provide lectures and assist in the training of nurses in end-of-life care. Many requests continue to be made to use the CARES tool for end-of-life education and training at other facilities throughout the United States and Canada. It provided a focus for the end-of-life house-wide initiatives developed at Sunnybrook Health Sciences Centre in Toronto, Canada, which is shared in Chapters 22 and 23.

Caring for the dying and their families can be one of the most emotionally fulfilling, personalized, and loving acts a nurse can provide. As Dr. Timothy Quill (1996) noted, the skills required to care for the dying are not high tech, but they are definitely high touch. The care nurses provide the dying and their families can change us as nurses and as human beings. Nurses can learn what is truly important in life and cannot help but be moved by the expressions of love and loss they will witness. The ability to empathize and provide compassionate care ultimately spills over into our daily interactions. It is common that nurses begin to view coworkers, their own families, and even the occasional angry car driver differently. They learn to embrace what is really important.

I hope to instill a sense of importance and urgency in the readers of this book. There is much to learn about providing quality evidence-based care for the dying and their families. This book about the CARES tool is unique in this regard as it attempts to convey essential information on how to effectively care for the dying in a condensed and readily applicable format for the bedside nurse. Stories and examples are provided to emphasize the importance of the nursing care required to effectively manage this much underserved growing population.

Quality evidence-based care of the dying is a special skill and can be developed and improved on with knowledge and experience. Additionally, nurses need to support each other and accept this very great challenge given to us by our aging society. Death must be accepted as a fact of life and honored. It is my hope that the use of the CARES tool will provide some guidance with this effort.

The chapters of this book help to dissect the CARES tool and show in detail the basis for its development and its many applications. Each chapter contributes to an example scenario about Steven, an actively dying 20-year-old young man with lymphocytic leukemia, whose treatment course was complicated by the development of graft-versus-host disease of the lung after bone marrow transplant. A basic overview of chapter content includes:

- A general background and the establishment of the CARES tool are found in Chapters 1 to 5.
- A detailed breakdown of the CARES tool by sections (comfort, airway, restlessness and delirium, emotional and spiritual support, and self-care) is discussed in Chapters 6 to 11.
- The theoretical foundation of the CARES tool is shared in Chapter 12.
- The need for patient advocacy and strong communication skills is emphasized in Chapters 13 and 14.
- Chapters 15 and 16 explore what can be done to promote a peaceful death, and case studies are provided.
- Chapters 17 and 18 address the changes in our culture that must occur and the new role of the doctor of nursing practice (DNP).
- Chapters 19 through 21 examine how the use of the CARES tool can impact nursing care and encourage end-of-life care involvement by other health care providers, and how hope can be nurtured for the dying.
- Chapters 22 and 23 provide insight into CARES tool application strategies employed at Sunnybrook Health Sciences Centre in Toronto, Canada.
- Chapter 24 summarizes the example scenario of Steven's final journey and the individualized care he and his family were given in an effort to provide a peaceful and loving death.
- Chapter 25 provides some recommended websites, readings, and references to continue the reader's education on evidence-based compassionate care of the dying.

Hospice, palliative care, and end-of-life care are complex medical specialties. The CARES tool does not provide a complete listing of all symptom management needs that could occur for the dying and their families. It attempts to address the most common issues encountered during the dying process. The CARES tool can only be fully understood and embraced as standard practice if additional end-of-life education is obtained. Ultimately, it is hoped that the CARES tool will empower nurses and health care staff to act as strong patient advocates, improve communication, provide individualized family-driven care, and employ the greatest gifts they have to offer a dying person and his or her family: the gift of their presence and their humanity (Puchalski & Ferrell, 2010).

In an effort to make the content of the CARES tool more accessible, a smartphone download is now available from Springer Publishing Company with the purchase of this book. Please visit http://www.springerpub.com/ compassionate-person-supplemental-materials to access this material.

Ultimately, the CARES tool was designed to address methods to help health care staff reduce if not eliminate the many treatable causes of suffering that can occur during the dying process. I close with Dr. Ira Byock's (2012) haunting observation that motivated me to develop the CARES tool:

> There are worse things than having someone you love die. Most basic, there is having the person you love die badly, suffering as he or she dies. Worse still is realizing later on that much of his or her suffering was unnecessary. (Preface)

Bonnie Freeman

REFERENCES

Byock, I. (2012). *The best care possible: A physician's quest to transform care through end of life.* New York, NY: Avery.

Freeman, B. (2013). CARES: An acronym organized tool for the care of the dying. *Journal of Hospice and Palliative Nursing, 15*(3), 147–153.

Puchalski, C. M., & Ferrell, B. R. (2010). *Making healthcare whole: Integrating spirituality into patient care.* West Conshohocken, PA: Templeton Press.

Quill, T. E. (1996). *A midwife through the dying process: Stories of healing & hard choices at the end of life.* Baltimore, MD: Johns Hopkins University Press.

Prologue: Reflections on End-of-Life Care

Death was an all too common outcome in the critical care units where I worked for the majority of my nursing career. I did not know that my desire to comfort and console the dying and their families would become a specialty form of care for me in the future. I believed it was just part of my nursing role to emotionally comfort individuals under my care and their families. The time I took to listen, allow individuals to speak of their fears, and sit quietly holding their hand was as important to me as any procedure or technical task. I simply gravitated to the care of the dying and their families, and was humbled and honored by the opportunity to help.

I believe the greatest training I obtained about caring for the dying came from the personal perspective I gained from caring for my parents and family as my mother died. I became acutely aware of how nurses interacted with the dying and their families during the death of my 48-year-old mother from lymphoma in 1986. I was 26 years old and a new nurse. I was totally naive when it came to caring for the dying; it was never discussed in nursing school, and I had no exposure to the specific skills that would be required. Unfortunately, I soon learned firsthand what not to do, and received my first life experience of how it felt to be abandoned, treated as insignificant, devalued, and ignored.

My mother was placed in a back hall, farthest from the nurse's station so as not to upset anyone while she was actively dying. Any call to the nurse's station for help was met with exasperated sighs, and then silence. I will always remember the overwhelming sense of helplessness, sadness, and loss that accompanied my mother's dying process. I remember an agitated respiratory therapist who informed me and my family that any further suctioning to decrease the bloody oral secretions produced by my mother would "just make her die faster," and that we "needed to stop calling because others that were more healthy need help."

I remember the oncologist who insisted he could still "cure" my mother—now with metastasis to the brain, bone, liver, kidneys, and lungs; with one blown pupil, unresponsive, and having Cheyne–Stokes respiration. How he begged my father and me not to "give up" on my mother, and how furious he was when we made her a do not resuscitate (DNR) and refused transfer to the intensive care unit. The oncologist angrily told my father and me that we were "killing her," and refused any further involvement in my mother's care.

My family and I wished only for our mother to die peacefully. It would have been so comforting to have had just one nurse take the time to be with us. I knew nothing more could be done, but recognized a deep need to know that someone else cared. We needed someone to sit and listen, to acknowledge our fears and pain, and to provide some small acts of compassion so we didn't feel so alone and abandoned. We needed someone to acknowledge our suffering and somehow validate our loss.

The lack of compassion and humanity caused me to feel like I was nothing and that my mother was nothing, and that none of us mattered. I will always remember the overwhelming grief and fear that I would never stop crying. I remember wondering how the nurses could ignore our suffering, and that they just didn't seem to care. It was the first time in my short career as a nurse that I was ashamed of my profession.

This personal experience motivated me to vow I would never allow a dying individual under my care or his or her family experience what I had endured. I believe it would have taken so little to make a difference. The emotional impact of having someone you love die before you is painful beyond words, and the abandonment I experienced during the last hours of my mother's life will forever be embedded in my memory.

This personal life experience motivated me to become the kind of nurse I wished had been there for me. Now, with each opportunity to comfort and assist a dying individual and his or her family, a personal healing takes place for me.

The development of the CARES tool was an extension of my vow. I began to realize that nurses were not intentionally distant or unfeeling when it came to caring for the dying; they just didn't know what to do. The CARES tool was developed to assist in providing this needed information in an easily accessible form, and to stimulate a desire to learn more about care of the dying. I continue to encourage nurses and anyone involved in the care of the dying to seek additional training from programs such as the End-of-Life Nursing Education Consortium (ELNEC).

I am humbled and honored by the opportunity to make a difference in the lives of the families of the dying, and have now found additional joy helping nurses improve their end-of-life care.

Bonnie Freeman

I had the pleasure of being introduced to Bonnie through my role as colead for the Quality Dying Initiative (QDI) at Sunnybrook Health Sciences Centre (SHSC), in Toronto, Ontario, Canada. In our organization, we decided that it was imperative for us to pay very close attention to the quality of the dying experience for all persons throughout the hospital. Through the QDI, we began our journey to positively transform care of the dying. Our first specific action was to design and implement a "Comfort Measures Strategy" across the hospital. In our search for an evidence-based approach to form the foundation of our change, we learned about the CARES tool and had the wonderful fortune to join forces with Bonnie.

By profession, I am a specialized oncology nurse and have been actively involved in cancer care for over 20 years, fulfilling various roles, including frontline nurse and leadership roles such as educator, professional leader, advanced practice nurse, and now director. These roles have enabled me to work in different settings, including the hospital, ambulatory care, and the community. This has further enhanced my understanding of end-of-life care, the diversity of patient and family needs, and the system barriers we face. I am so grateful for the privilege of living my passion as a nurse. Being present with individuals and their families through their personal health journeys has changed me and caused me to continuously reflect on what I believe and what I know. It has challenged me to live my own life differently, and to strive to find ways to improve the experience of health care from the perspectives of those we care for.

End of life is an inevitable point in the journey for all of us as human beings. And yet it remains an aspect of care that is challenging, elusive, and often silent. I am keenly aware that I bring to my nursing role all my past experiences caring for those who have died, and my own personal story. In my life, I have been significantly impacted through the deaths of those whom I love: my father, uncles, mother-in-law, and father-in-law. Each of their journeys was very different, and each revealed new insights and learning that have been woven into my life and have further driven my commitment to influence change.

As a daughter, I sat silently by the side of my father in an intensive care unit, after having his ventilator removed, watching his erratic breathing, waiting and wondering if each breath would be his last. I know how it feels to wait, to feel pain and sadness, to not know when it will come to an end, to hope for death and not want it, all at the same time. I know that when it is said that there is "nothing more that can be done," we have limited our meaning of caring. There is so much more that can be done. We must recognize that caring in itself provides comfort and hope, and often the greatest gifts are the simplest gestures that are long remembered.

Tracey Das Gupta

My first exposure to caring for individuals who were facing death and their family members was as a new clinical nurse specialist in the mid-1970s. Oncology was just emerging as a specialty, and a large majority of those who were diagnosed with cancer died following rather arduous courses of therapy fraught with numerous side-effect management issues. This was before the advent of effective antiemetic therapies and other supportive care medications. Death was not often discussed openly, and palliative care as a philosophy had not yet entered the realm of clinical practice in our environment.

I was invited as a nursing practice consultant by the oncology team, to help the staff nurses cope with the challenges they were feeling as they cared for individuals who were dying on their unit. The nurses talked of challenges in having conversations, feeling tensions between quality-of-life and quantity-of-life goals for care, dealing with the myriad side effects the dying were experiencing, and handling the various wishes of everyone involved in the situation. They found it particularly difficult when the dying and their family members did not agree on a specific course of action or plan of care. At the time, one of the biggest issues was having an open conversation about DNR orders—there was no precedent for having this type of conversation or for coming to consensus as a team about what was to be done. Frequently, patients were not informed clearly about their diagnosis, let alone their prognosis; and the idea of actually consulting the patient about his or her wishes was not really considered. On reflection, it was a challenging time.

But for me, this was the beginning and it has been a long but rewarding journey since then. Over the years, I have had the opportunity to learn about palliative and end-of-life care, its philosophy and approach, and see the evidence for the field grow. I have had the chance to work closely with Canadian leaders in this field, to drive policy and program change, and to engage in the education of nurses about end-of-life care. It has been wonderful to participate in the introduction and feel part of the growth of the field over the years. I was thrilled recently to see that it is now acknowledged as a clinical specialty in Canada, and access to palliative care service is now stated as a standard of quality patient care and a hallmark of a high-performing health system.

I saw evidence that the field had grown when my own father died of cancer. He was informed of his diagnosis and prognosis and given choices about what he wanted to do. The actions taken by the health care team members that allowed him to spend quality time at home were so meaningful. His side effects were managed according to his wishes and the current state of knowledge about them. And my mother and the family members were included in the dialogue and decision making with him. The experience also left me with a clear picture of the difference between being a health professional in the field, when you think you have command and control, and suddenly being thrust into the reality of being a daughter and losing a loved one. Without a doubt, the conversations the staff members had with us as family members, the openness of their support, and the way I observed how they cared for Dad made all the difference in my experience then and my remembrances of that difficult time.

Margaret Fitch

PART I

Care for the Dying

CHAPTER 1

Introduction to the CARES Tool

In 2012, a very skilled and respected oncologist, Dr. Chatchada Karanes, MD, sought my assistance as a palliative care nurse practitioner (NP) to help a 20-year-old male and his family through the dying process. This was not a routine request at the 300-bed cancer research facility where I worked, as most palliative care consults were strictly for pain management. The need and perceived value of palliative care consults were in their infancy, and end-of-life (EOL) consults were extremely rare. Resistance to a change in culture that incorporates palliative care was not unique to my hospital as they maintained the traditional curative focus held nationally in the United States.

Death remained an unacceptable outcome, an admission of failure, and a tragic response. Only a few physicians were beginning to view death as a possible consequence of a disease process to be supported and achieved peacefully after curative treatment was no longer an option and life-prolonging measures were deemed futile. Death in a cancer facility was just beginning to be viewed as a part of life and not exclusively as a failure.

The exceptional reputation of Dr. Karanes made her request all the more flattering, and I was genuinely impressed by her acceptance of the inevitable death of this young man under her care and her desire for his death to be as compassionate and as peaceful as possible. She welcomed my assistance to address his final stage of life and viewed EOL care as important as any other acute care procedure. I was grateful that the message of support and desire to assist in providing personalized and family-specific symptom management was being heard.

STEVEN'S STORY

The young man I was asked to see was diagnosed with acute lymphocytic leukemia and had undergone a bone marrow transplant 3 months ago. He developed an all too common complication of this treatment called graft-versus-host disease. This often-aggressive disease process was attacking his lungs. The leukemia was in remission, but the cost was a progressive and irreversible loss of lung function. This otherwise healthy young man was now slowly suffocating. Dr. Karanes asked me to provide whatever comfort I could for this actively dying young man and his family and not allow them to suffer.

In the role of a pain and palliative care NP, providing EOL care for individuals and their families was an important aspect of the services provided by the palliative care team. This role should not be exclusive to palliative care NPs as they continue to be the primary caregivers and are in a position to make an enormous impact on the lives of the dying and on a grieving family. It requires very little technical skill. The needed care is so basic, it is often overlooked or deemed unimportant. How could just being present and listening, offering a cup of tea to a family member, or applying a warm washcloth to the forehead of someone who is dying make any difference? It is my hope the readers of this book will find that the nurse's acts of compassion and humanity will provide a huge difference. The specific act is often forgotten by the family member, but the implied meaning is retained. Yes, the washcloth or a cup of tea is insignificant, but the meaning behind them demonstrates respect, a desire to comfort, an acknowledgment of the value of the individual, and a sense of compassion that will positively support the grieving family members. If the memory of a loved one's death is perceived as loving, calm, and supportive because of a nurse's compassionate actions, the grieving process can be greatly assisted. This additional support will be invaluable for years to come as the family members struggle to find peace and acceptance of their loss. If the memory of a loved one's death is filled with emotional pain, abandonment, and doubt, grieving can actually be intensified. This emotional trauma was identified as a contributing factor for the development of posttraumatic stress for one out of three family members that experience a perceived unsupported death (Ferrell & Coyle, 2010). The emotional trauma will impact that family member for the rest of his or her life and could result in the development of multiple psychiatric and socially dysfunctional behaviors.

Numerous terminally ill individuals and their families have expressed concerns about the dying process. The fear of pain and suffering is what frightened these individuals the most. Often, death itself was not the focus of their fears as much as *how* they would die. It is the "how" that remains responsible for the greatest anxiety. Families worry about their loved one suffering, and terminally ill persons worry about their family being supported and not feeling abandoned or overcome with grief. Dr. Ira Byock (2012) expressed the importance of obtaining evidence-based knowledge on the care of the dying when he claimed that in this time of technology and resources there are no excuses for allowing the dying or their family to suffer. This is a deeply held belief within palliative medicine, and demonstrates the commitment I felt to assist this dying young man and his family through their final journey together.

The name of the young man was Steven. Soon after the consult request, I visited Steven and assessed how he was progressing. On arrival to his unit, I encountered three very anxious nurses and Nicole, a very caring and experienced social worker, trying to help. The nurses informed me that Steven was actively dying. My heart ached when I first met Steven. He was an emaciated, pale, and diaphoretic young man who appeared five times his age. His bald head and withered body were positioned upright on pillows. His mother was sitting on a chair next to his bed rubbing his arm with a gloved hand. She was gowned and gloved, just like the protective isolation sign instructed. Her green eyes were now red and swollen as her tears continued to flow into her white cotton mask. Steven had the same green eyes but his were open wide as he stared blankly at the ceiling. His respirations were agonal, coming at irregular intervals as his shoulders and upper chest heaved in a spasm-like motion with each breath. His pressurized oxygen mask system (BiPAP) hissed in its effort to force oxygen into Steven's rigid lungs.

A middle-aged man with a heavily wrinkled yellow isolation gown approached the health care providers from a corner chair where he sat away from Steven's bed. Everyone introduced themselves and I found out that the gentleman was Steven's father. He looked exhausted and his voice trembled when he spoke as he struggled to maintain emotional control. The first question he asked me was, "Do you think he is suffering?"

I found many nurses hesitate to answer this commonly asked question. Nursing schools do not routinely prepare nurses to interact with the dying and their families, nor do they provide an emphasis on the need to communicate effectively. I realized how badly the nurses wanted to help, and how unprepared they were. Based on this observation and the experience with Steven, I planned to develop a teaching tool that could help nurses provide compassionate evidence-based care for the dying in the form of a quick reference guide.

I designed the tool to draw on the scholarly works of such knowledgeable experts in the field of palliative care as Betty Ferrell, RN, PhD, MA, FAAN, FPCN; Christine Puchalski, MD; Ira Byock, MD; Timothy Quill,

MD; Nessa Coyle, PhD, APRN, FAAN; and Elaine Wittenberg-Lyles, PhD, and wanted to instill a new respect for the skills required to effectively care for the dying by using an acronym format to encourage an association with other acronym-based programs such as BCLS (basic cardiac life support) and ACLS (advanced cardiac life support).

I decided to do a literature review and identify the most frequently addressed symptom management needs of the dying. The review indicated pain, respiratory distress, delirium, and emotional and spiritual distress to be the most common. The literature review also identified the need for self-care for health care providers caring for the dying.

I consolidated the five most common EOL care needs into a reference guide organized by the acronym CARES.

- The "C" was selected to represent the need for comfort. This included both pain management and general comfort measures.
- The "A" was selected to represent measures to address airway management. It involved the need to treat respiratory distress, provide secretion control, and make suggestions for educating family members on the breathing changes commonly seen with the dying.
- The "R" was used to designate the restlessness commonly observed with the dying; more accurately termed delirium.
- The "E" was selected to represent the emotional issues common to the dying and their families. Spirituality was included in this section to allow for a more holistic focus for the kind of support commonly required.
- The "S" addressed the newest focus of concern when caring for the dying: self-care, to address the impact death can have on the caregiver.

The CARES tool was designed to address EOL care knowledge deficits and assist the bedside nurse to more fully understand the unique care required during the dying process. It encourages nurses to act as advocates for dying individuals and their families, and to tailor their care to their specific needs (see Exhibits 1.1–1.5).

The CARES tool was designed to help nurses in situations similar to the one under current discussion about Steven. Without training and experience, a nurse placed in this position would be challenged to provide the kind of physical and emotional support needed to answer questions about suffering, and assist an individual, such as Steven, to die in comfort.

The needs of Steven and his family are extensive. There is much that can be done to make Steven's death a loving and peaceful experience for him, his family, and the nursing staff caring for him. Education and experience help nurses to better understand the needs of the dying. Training is essential for nurses to provide the unique care that is required. The CARES tool attempts to summarize this care and encourages nurses to take on the much needed role of advocate. Nurses are in a unique position to improve the quality of care provided for all dying individuals by

EXHIBIT 1.1 Comfort section of the CARES tool.

Comfort

You must act as an advocate for your patient to control his or her pain. Pain control is an essential need for all dying patients.

- The route of the medication determines time to maximum effect:
  - IV peak effect is 15 minutes ¬ Orally in 60 minutes
  - Sub-q in 30 minutes ¬ Transdermal 6–8 hours
- Terminal pain/pain during dying is best managed by around-the-clock, scheduled, or a continuous infusion of opioid (such as from a PCA pump) and additional doses (boluses) given as needed for breakthrough pain.
- There is no maximum dose of opioids for pain control.
- Nurses are often frightened that the opioid they give a patient will cause him or her to die prematurely.
  - There will always be a last dose when caring for a dying patient. Keep in mind the legal and ethical concepts of intent.
  - The patient is dying because of his or her disease process, not the opioid.
- Adjustments in dosage or type of opioid may be required in the presence of renal failure, and if the pain medication does not help to control the patient's pain.
  - Consider fentanyl if the patient has renal failure and if the patient has small seizure-like tremors (myoclonus).
  - Opioids stay in the system longer in case of renal failure. Dosage is usually smaller.
  - Consider changing the type of opiate if pain remains uncontrolled.

The focus of care for the dying patient is comfort. All unnecessary procedures, tests, and activities should be evaluated. Providing as much time for the patient and his or her family to be together should be the priority. Consider obtaining orders as appropriate for the following:

- Stop or modify vital signs
- Stop oral medications if unable to swallow and all nonessential medications
- Clarify IV options: stop or reduce
- Stop or reduce tube feedings
- Turn off monitors and alarms
- Stop or decrease labs per physician and family preference
- Discontinue isolation

You can provide the following comfort measures without an order:

- Turn and position patient only for comfort
- Modify bathing or stop per family request
- Consider reinforcing dressings only
- Provide frequent oral care
- Provide oral suctioning if family requests
- Provide temperature comfort measures such as a cool washcloth and ice packs
- Explain mottling and cyanosis as part of the dying process and not from being cold

EXHIBIT 1.2 Airway section of the CARES tool.

Airway

The use of supplemental oxygen during the dying process is often ineffective but may help to minimize the family's fears of their loved one suffering. Review goals of care established by the patient and family for supplemental O_2.

- Consider use of a fan
- Provide nasal cannula per MD orders
- Reposition patient as needed

The dying process results in irregular breathing with periods of apnea. Secretions often pool in the back of the patient's throat resulting in loud congestive sounds. Patients can become restless and anxious. Consider obtaining orders for:

- Glycopyrrolate, scopolamine patch, or atropine 1% ophthalmic solution
- Morphine IV or Sub-q: The patient is dying and will stop breathing due to his or her disease and the dying process, and not from receiving morphine
- Consider using antianxiety agents and/or antipsychotics

Provide family education as needed; some common issues to address are:

- Breathing patterns of the dying. Breathing becomes progressively irregular, shallow, and slowed. Episodes of apnea will extend. This is all from brain stem activity. It is involuntary and the patient is not suffering.
- Emphasize the calming effects of touch and talking to the patient

---

EXHIBIT 1.3 Restlessness and delirium section of the CARES tool.

Restlessness and Delirium

The restlessness that commonly occurs during the dying process is also called terminal or agitated delirium. It can also result from pain, bladder distention, or stool impaction. The patient must be protected from injury and the family needs to be supported. Consider the following:

- Give a trial dose of opioids to rule out pain
- Assess for bladder distention and insert indwelling catheter if needed
- Assess for impaction if appropriate
- Consider antipsychotics: haloperidol or chlorpromazine
- Consider benzodiazepines: lorazepam or midazolam
- Maintain calm environment
- Minimize bright lights
- Play patient's favorite music
- Talk softly to patient; maintain use of touch and presence
- Comfort patient by saying: "You are safe. We are with you. We love you."
- Consider aromatherapy

Unfinished business may cause restlessness. Discuss with the family possible causes of anxiety.

- Review with the family the importance of saying good-bye and giving permission to stop fighting
- Question family about an important family event or anniversary

Educate the family on:

- Patient lacking awareness of behavior
- Possibility of being peacefully confused

EXHIBIT 1.4 Emotional and spiritual support section of the CARES tool.

Emotional and Spiritual Support

Providing emotional, spiritual, psychosocial, and cultural support to the patient and family allows us to care for the soul. This is the very foundation of caring for the dying. It is important to know your resources:

- Notify supportive care medicine team members for assistance. Be specific if resources are for patient, staff, or both.
- Always work to retain the patient's dignity and feelings of value.
- Remember every family is unique and grieves differently. Good communication is essential:
  - Ensure communication exists with the family and all disciplines.
  - Take your cues from the family. Do not assume you know what they are thinking or feeling
  - Clarify how much the family wants to know
  - Clarify goals of care
  - Clarify privacy needs
- Just be with patient and family and sit in silence
- Work with family to provide favorite activities, smells, sounds, etc.
- Support rituals and assist with obtaining desired clergy or equipment.

Other activities and methods of support to consider:
- Your humanity is needed the most now. Always be available. Your very presence is reassuring to the family.
- The family is an important part of your patient care and becomes your focus as the patient becomes more unresponsive.
  - Be sure families are getting rest and breaks
  - Provide coffee, water, etc.
  - Continue to be available to answer questions
  - You cannot take away their pain; acknowledge their emotion and be present
- Play a patient's favorite music.
- Position the bed to see out a window.
- Encourage the family to provide patient's favorite hat, clothing, etc.
- Lower or mute lighting.
- Consider bringing in favorite pet.

EXHIBIT 1.5 Self-care section of the CARES tool.

Self-Care

The health care providers must allow themselves to be human and expect some personal emotional response to the death of their patient and for the grieving family. Palliative/supportive services are available to staff. Often, a review and debriefing can assist with professional grieving and promote emotional health by:

- Recognizing the stressful event and thanking supportive team members
- Reviewing what went well and what challenges need to be addressed
- Sharing comments of the bereaved family
- Addressing moral distress issues
- Expressing issues of death anxiety and obtaining support
- Exploring challenges and privileges of assisting a fellow human being through the dying process
- Acknowledging the spiritual impact of witnessing death
- Exploring how your care made a difference to the grieving family
- Reviewing effective communication techniques, available resources, and support

championing the delivery of evidence-based compassionate EOL care as a standard of practice.

This book attempts to supply additional information and insight into the important role nurses need to embrace when caring for the dying. It provides information about the CARES tool and offers further rationale to explain the prompts and suggestions furnished in the tool for consideration.

The CARES tool emphasizes:

1. Care of dying individuals must include methods to address their specific needs and those of their families.

2. All dying individuals and their families have unique methods of grieving, communication, and holistic supportive needs.

3. The dying person and his or her family must be treated as one unit.

4. The need for the nurse to develop good teaching skills and effective communication techniques to provide individualized, empathetic, and compassionate holistic care.

5. The need for nurses to be advocates for individuals under their care through clear communication of mutually established goals, anticipation of necessary medications, equipment, and treatment adjustments, and holistically supporting a peaceful death.

6. The need for nurses to embrace the importance of their humanity, compassion, empathy, ability to actively listen, and to be therapeutically present.

7. The importance of self-care, professional grieving, and the need to acknowledge and address the impact caring for the dying has on us as human beings.

Basic tools and rationale on how to achieve the goals addressed in the CARES tool are provided throughout the chapters of this book.

The CARES tool is supported by extensive peer-reviewed literature on care of the dying. The volumes of evidence-based information can be overwhelming and often intimidating when a bedside nurse just wants to know what to do next. The CARES tool is based on the most common needs of the dying and their families identified in the literature and arranged in an acronym format. The busy nurse can quickly review what still needs to be addressed and what they can request or order within their scope of practice. A strong background based in education and training for the dying is essential for the most effective use of the CARES tool.

It is also essential that a nurse caring for a dying individual is aware of his or her own cultural and spiritual beliefs, and concerns about death. If a fear or concern about some aspect of the dying process exists, it is common for the nurse to withdraw in an unconscious effort for self-protection. Nurses must become aware of their feelings and reactions toward death.

Nurses cannot help but bring their uncertainties or cultural bias to the bedside, but they can be tempered if one is self-aware.

A positive focus on caring for the dying must also be noted as many nurses and health care professionals enjoy this challenging discipline of health care. Hospice nurses continue to demonstrate low job turnover rates often recounting amazement about how much they receive personally with each caring experience. Hospice nurses express an awareness of the opportunity to rework personal losses, an ability to more easily dismiss inconveniences and irritations, an acute awareness of the beauty that exists around them, and a deep appreciation of life because of their interactions with the terminally ill.

The dying and their families have so much they can teach us, and nurses have so much they can give. When a balance is achieved, the interaction can be deeply spiritual. Nurses are challenged by the dying to help them feel respected, valued, supported, and listened to in the fast-paced computerized hospital setting. Acting in this compassionate and humanistic manner will help keep many nurses grounded and focused on what is really important. They will be reminded that the greatest gifts they can provide the dying and their families are their willingness to actively listen, educate, reassure, empathize, compassionately communicate and, above all, embrace the use of their humanity.

The needs of the dying are the reasons many individuals become nurses and the care they require mirrors what nurses identify as what differentiates them from any other health care professional. It is time nurses embrace their role as advocates and honor the unique services only they can provide. Nurses are trained to care holistically and advocating the needs of persons under their care is essential to this role.

REFERENCES

Byock, I. (2012). *The best care possible: A physician's quest to transform care through end of life*. New York, NY: Avery.

Ferrell, B. R., & Coyle, N. (Eds.). (2010). *Oxford textbook of palliative nursing* (3rd ed.). New York, NY: Oxford University Press.

CHAPTER 2

History of Caring for the Dying

DeSpelder and Strickland (2015) in their book, *The Last Dance: Encountering Death and Dying*, noted the Italian philosopher Giambattista Vico's observation that the Latin root word for humanity is *humare*, which means to bury. It is often our very humanity that is lacking in our care of the dying. It is our kindness and compassion that are required to assist the dying and their families through their final journey together. This is the ultimate role that demonstrates our humanity.

Our humanity requires that death be honored and revered as it is in many cultures. Death is viewed as a stage of transition to a higher level of functioning, a beginning closely equated with birth, and as difficult to discern as a sunrise from a sunset. Death is celebrated as a grateful acknowledgment of the gift of time spent with the now deceased. Our very humanity was established in this celebration of a life well lived, and of the individual that would be deeply missed.

Death in the 1900s continued to be a normal part of life. Life expectancy was only 47 years. Eighty percent of the population died at home after a very short period of illness or injury, and the family was the dominate caregiver (DeSpelder & Strickland, 2015; Ferrell & Coyle, 2010). In 2011, only 20% of all Americans died at home, 30% died in extended care facilities, and 50% died in hospitals (Byock, 2012).

World War I (1914–1918) brought new technology, and the medicalization of dying (DeSpelder & Strickland, 2015). More individuals began dying in hospitals. Dying became a private event as it moved away from the community. Professionals dictated care, usurping the role of the family and close friends, implying that their incompetence and inability could not meet the needs of the dying. Strangers now imposed standardized management of the dying that was considered "professional" by the local culture. The decision to hide all signs of death and dying from society marked the beginning of what was termed "invisible death" in our culture (DeSpelder & Strickland, 2015).

As technology grew, death evolved into a secretive dark place that no one wanted to acknowledge. Care of the dying did not keep pace with this new technology. Advances in care of the dying stagnated in this progressive curative culture. Death became a disease to be conquered and managed. It was associated with failure, a mistake, a punishment from God, and something to be ignored or made less visible (DeSpelder & Strickland, 2015).

Soon, it was no longer acceptable to have a funeral in the parlor of the home. Parlors were renamed living rooms to deny that death ever came into a home. Death needed to be kept separate from the living. When grandpa died in his bed, his body was immediately moved to the local funeral home; the only remaining place where death was allowed. Funeral homes worked to make the body of the deseased as life-like as possible, so families could console themselves with the illusion that grandpa was only sleeping.

Even the words death and dying were rarely spoken out loud. In many cases, alternative phrases were used that soften or mute the fact that death has occurred. Similar sayings continue to this day, such as he or she passed away, went on to their final reward, are finally at peace, caught the bus, bought the farm, or simply are no longer with us. Avoiding all discussions about dying is common in our culture, but as the population continues to age, death is becoming more of a reality we will all one day embrace. With aging comes the eventual inability to deny our mortality.

This gradual awareness of the need to improve care of the dying resulted in the acceptance of the work of Dame Cicely Saunders and prompted her to visit Yale University's School of Nursing in 1963. In 1966, the dean of Yale's graduate nursing program, Florence Wald, organized a meeting with Saunders, Elisabeth Kübler-Ross, Colin Murray Parkes, and others in the field of dying and was instrumental in establishing the hospice movement in America. The first hospice in the United States was established in 1974, in New Haven, Connecticut.

Hospitals soon identified the need to establish hospice-like programs within their facilities and the first hospital-based palliative care team was established at St. Luke's Hospital in New York City in 1974. Palliative care was utilized to address the holistic symptom management needs of the chronically ill and to provide this same supportive care needed by individuals not eligible for hospice (life prognosis of 6 months or less). A focus was established on quality of life and the belief that there is always something that can be offered to the dying even if curative treatment is not an option. There is a need to assist the terminally ill to live a full life as they define it until their death (DeSpelder & Strickland, 2015). This care must continue to address the psychological, social, emotional, and spiritual needs of the terminally ill and their families and not just the physical.

In the 1990s, the increasing awareness of our mortality and the effectiveness of home hospice programs resulted in an increased demand for palliative care as many baby boomers resolved they would not die in darkness and suffer as their parents did. There was a growing effort to reintroduce compassion and holistic care back into the sterile world of technical advances that was removing all sense of humanity from medical management. The paternal role of the physician was giving way to the push for autonomy and a right for the individual to voice an opinion about his or her care. Those terminally ill and their families wanted a part in the decision-making process to decide what treatments they would undergo, to define what quality of life meant to them, and to be treated with dignity and respect.

The hospice movement provided a compassionate example of what death could be and supported the hospital-based initiative to provide the same quality of care (Ferrell & Coyle, 2010). Palliative care teams and educated health care staff were trained to acknowledge the suffering of individuals and families and help to transcend emotional burdens through empathy, active listening, dignity-affirming therapies, and demonstrating and promoting respect. This specialized education and training is not furnished as part of a standard health care provider's academic program. Without this education and experience, meeting the needs of the dying and their families is problematic as resources are not recognized or consulted and necessary spiritual and psychosocial support is not provided (Puchalski & Ferrell, 2010).

Individuals continue to die in pain today because health care providers remain uneducated regarding effective pain management (Bookbinder et al., 2005; Brajtman, 2005). Health care providers are hesitant to effectively treat the pain of the dying because of concerns over accelerating the dying process, addiction, and fears of euthanasia. Relieving pain and eliminating suffering are the intent and can actually prolong life. Promoting quality continues to be the necessary focus of end-of-life (EOL) care. The understanding of these concepts can only occur with education and experience (Thurston, Wilson, & Hewitt, 2011).

It is becoming more apparent that care of the dying is much more than just care of the body. To help facilitate a peaceful death, health care providers must also learn to care for the soul (Puchalski & Ferrell, 2010). This will require an emphasis on cultivating warm and accepting relationships with the dying and their families, developing extraordinary listening and communication skills, and striving to remove fears of abandonment and worthlessness (Puchalski & Ferrell, 2010). Caring for the soul means ". . . recognizing the power in our own humanity to make a difference in the lives of others and valuing it as highly as our expertise" (2010, p. xx).

Dickinson (2007) noted that the average amount of time expended on EOL care education in medical and nursing programs was 15 hours. Health care providers continue to express anxiety and difficulty in effectively addressing the needs of the dying. Mutto, Cantoni, Rabhanansi, and Villar (2011) stated that health care professionals considered their basic education on care of the dying to be woefully inadequate. Currently practicing health care providers are providing care for the dying often without any EOL training (Sanchez-Reilly & Ross, 2012).

Care of the actively dying hospitalized individual varies based on the expertise of the nursing staff, involvement of a palliative care team, the timeliness of enacting comfort measures, the presence and honoring of advance directives, and the early initiation of clear communication to confirm and support the individual and his or her family's goals of care (Wittenberg-Lyles, Goldsmith, & Ragan, 2011). In a study by Becker et al. (2007), the average initiation of comfort care plans occurred 9 days prior to death, one third of the dying continued to receive active life-sustaining treatment until death, and the prognosis of dying was made 3.8 days prior to death. Of the terminally ill individuals, 50% will die in pain, and 80% of the dying will experience suboptimally treated dyspnea and terminal restlessness or delirium before they die (LeGrand & Walsh, 2011; Ong, Yee, & Lee, 2012).

REFERENCES

Becker, G., Sarhatlic, R., Olschewski, M., Xander, C., Momm, F., & Blum, H. E. (2007). End-of-life care in hospital: Current practice and potentials for improvement. *Journal of Pain and Symptom Management, 33*(6), 711–719.

Bookbinder, M., Blank, A. E., Arney, E., Wollner, D., Lesage., P., McHugh, M., Portenoy, R. K. (2005). Improving end of life care: Development and pilot-test of a clinical pathway. *Journal of Pain and Symptom Management, 29*(6), 529–543.

Brajtman, S. (2005). Helping the family through the experience of terminal restlessness. *Journal of Hospice and Palliative Nursing, 7*(2), 73–81.

Byock, I. (2012). *The best care possible: A physician's quest to transform care through end of life.* New York, NY: Avery.

DeSpelder, L. A., & Strickland, A. L. (2015). *The last dance: Encountering death and dying* (10th ed.). New York, NY: McGraw-Hill.

Dickinson, G. (2007). End-of-life and palliative care issues in medical and nursing schools in the United States. *Death Studies, 31*(8), 713–726.

Ferrell, B. R., & Coyle, N. (Eds.). (2010). *Oxford textbook of palliative nursing* (3rd ed.). New York, NY: Oxford University Press.

LeGrand, S. B., & Walsh, D. (2011). Comfort measures: Practical care of the dying cancer patient. *American Journal of Hospice and Palliative Medicine, 27*(7), 488–493.

Mutto, E. M., Cantoni, M. N., Rabhanansi, M. M., & Villar, M. J. (2011). A perspective of end-of-life education in undergraduate medical and nursing students in Buenos Aires, Argentina. *Journal of Palliative Medicine, 15*(1), 93–98.

Ong, W., Yee, C. M., & Lee, A. (2012). Ethical dilemmas in the care of cancer patients near the end of life. *Singapore Medical Journal, 53*(1), 11–14.

Puchalski, C. M., & Ferrell, B. R. (2010). *Making health care whole: Integrating spiritually into practice* [Electronic Edition]. West Conshohocken, PA: Templeton Press.

Sanchez-Reilly, S., & Ross, J. S. (2012). Hospice and palliative medicine: Curriculum evaluation and learner assessment in medical education. *Journal of Palliative Medicine, 15*(1), 116–122.

Thurston, A. J., Wilson, D. M., & Hewitt, J. A. (2011). Current end-of-life care needs and care practices in acute care hospitals. *Nursing Research and Practice*, Article ID 869302, http://dx.doi.org/10.1155/2011/869302

Wittenberg-Lyles, E., Goldsmith, J., & Ragan, S. (2011). The shift to early palliative care: A typology of illness journeys and the role of nursing. *Clinical Journal of Oncology Nursing, 15*(3), 304–319.

CHAPTER 3

Goals and Objectives When Caring for the Dying

When caring for the dying, goals of care should always be developed based on individual and family preferences. Patients and their families have lost all control over the disease process, and any sense of control, whether it occurs with the ability to decide code status or if blood work will continue to be drawn, must be provided. Health care providers cannot begin to anticipate or appreciate the numerous losses these individuals are addressing. Priorities may often become unique during the final stages of the dying process. The most common goals for the dying and their families focus on the elimination of suffering, devising methods to ensure good communication, and respecting and supporting family rituals. Each dying experience is unique and should reflect the needs and desires of the persons involved. This can only occur with clear communication and an established rapport.

GOAL SETTING AND FAMILY DYNAMICS

Goal setting requires that individuals are comfortable expressing their feelings and any sense of being judged is removed. It is essential that the nurses not interject their personal priorities or expectations. The focus must be on what is important to the dying individual and his or her family. Often, our own priorities, biases, or habits prevent families from obtaining the closure they require. One of the most difficult goals for most nurses to understand is a family's desire not to be present as their loved one dies, or their request not to be called. Nurses must remember that family dynamics are unique. If a family is dysfunctional, they are very likely to become more dysfunctional under stress. This statement does not mean to imply that all family members who do not wish to be present at the death of their loved one are dysfunctional. There are many reasons for this decision, such as wishing to remember the individual as he or she once was, or feeling the emotion of the event would be too traumatic for them to handle publicly. As nurses, we are expected to act in the best interest of a person under our care and his or her family; his or her wishes should be respected. This can be challenging when we do not agree with a decision of an individual or a family member. Our obligation remains to ensure their decisions are fully informed and to advocate for their wishes.

GOAL SETTING THROUGH ACTIVE LISTENING

Information necessary to develop goals can only be acquired through active listening and encouraging the family to share their loved one's values and priorities. Often asking about interests and what the patient enjoys doing for relaxation and recreation is helpful. The information can assist to clearly define what "living" meant for the dying individual, and it provides the family an opportunity to remember and celebrate the person they love instead of focusing on their pending loss. The clear identification of a person's needs and desires also allows for a separation of his or her needs from those of his or her loved ones. Goal setting often allows for the identification of who is actually being taken care of, and very often it is not the individual who is dying. Family members once shared how their father would want everything possible done because he would never want to leave them. After closer examination it was discovered that a family member was the one who could not let go. Family members often require gentle redirection to identify whose needs are really being met. One nurse shared a statement to help with this concept. She noted that often the most loving act an individual will ever make or agree to will be the very one that will break his or her heart. She gave the example of giving your loved one permission to stop fighting, and telling him or her that you will be alright, all the while knowing that this statement is not true, but you want your dying loved one to stop worrying about you. When helped to realize what their actions or inactions may cause, many family members do not want their loved one to suffer and struggle just for them. The goal for the family member becomes one in which his or her loved one dies in peace.

GOAL SETTING THROUGH FOCUSING ON THE NEEDS AND DESIRES OF THE DYING INDIVIDUAL

When setting goals, it is important to be focused on the needs and desires of the dying individual. The dying are so much more than their disease, and they are no longer in a position to take care of their family's needs. Their life should be celebrated and it is time for the family to take care of them.

At a large family meeting for Mr. S, a 42-year-old divorced father of three, the family came together to discuss goals of care. There were 12 family members present at the meeting. The primary physician opened the meeting and discussed the status of Mr. S's aggressive renal cancer and the massive myocardial infarction and resultant liver failure that occurred as a complication of the chemotherapy. The family members were all visibly upset at the prospect of their loved one dying. The physician shared the concerns voiced by the dying man over what will happen to his family without him. The physician revealed how the man agonized over the thought of abandoning his children. After this statement was made, the tears and sobbing in the room abruptly stopped. The family realized they were grieving over the pending loss of this wonderful man and never considered what he may be feeling or needing. The goals of care shifted to celebrating and supporting Mr. S. Plans were made to bring in his favorite ball cap and blue jeans. The family decided they would savor the time they had and focus on quality time together.

It is common for families to require some gentle redirection as their personal needs are often interpreted as those of the dying. Nurses can help families set realistic goals of care if a focus is placed on what was important to the dying individual. Often, families need help to understand issues of futility, comfort, and quality of life versus prolonging the dying process.

Some common needs to address regarding concerns over the dying process include:

1. Viewing the dying person as an individual and not just a diagnosis
2. Retaining the person's dignity and feelings of being valued and comforted
3. Obtaining closure and a peaceful and loving way to say good-bye
4. Avoiding pain and suffering
5. Setting nursing goals

Nursing goals can be easily developed from the individual's and the family's goals of care. The translation could be as follows.

1. Always treat the individual under their care as unique and with respect
2. Provide individualized person-centered care
3. Encourage direct communication that promotes closure
4. Provide evidence-based quality symptom management

Specific objectives to meet the identified nursing goals can now be developed. Again, all objectives must be individual and family focused, and incorporate established goals of care. Some objectives utilizing the stated nursing goals may include:

1. Promote and maintain respect for the individual and his or her family as evidenced by knocking before entering his or her room, calling the person by his or her desired name, actively listening to the individual and his or her family, and seeking his or her input on decisions of care

2. Seek individual and family input on desired care, timing of procedures, and methods to achieve desired outcomes such as comfort, as it applies to positioning, choice of clothing, dressing changes, obtaining vital signs, and so on

3. Promote and maintain open communication as evidenced by family members' confirmation of understanding through the use of family meetings, and maintaining constant nurse availability for questions or concerns

4. Educate family on the dying process to enable them to differentiate between a normal dying process and suffering as evidenced by the family's verbalization of understanding

5. The need for an individualized plan of care

The need for an individualized plan of care is essential. The dying person and his or her family should feel there is a shared plan to achieve the goals of care. This becomes more challenging when addressing medical futility. When the individual you are caring for or a family member expresses a goal that is deemed physically and/or ethically unrealistic, therapeutic communication must occur. Risks versus benefits becomes the focal point of discussion, and ensuring information is provided that will result in an informed decision about care.

Special nursing skills are needed to address the final days to hours of life when all treatment options have been exhausted and comfort measures are the agreed course of action. Occasionally, families and some dying individuals will request one final treatment, surgery, or procedure in an attempt to buy more time. Goals of care should never imply withholding or taking away any treatment. They should be framed in such a way as to focus on what is being provided. This positive phrasing greatly assists the family to acknowledge everything possible is being done to provide comfort and support to their dying loved one. An example of this strategy could occur when a terminally ill person requests one more chemotherapy treatment and the physician knows the risks will far outweigh the benefits because the chemotherapy requested has already proven to be ineffective. Rather than refusing, further investigation is needed to establish the individual's perception of what he or she hopes to achieve by receiving one more chemotherapy treatment. If the individual admits he or she is just trying to buy more time, a dialogue could be established to include the risks and possible alterations to the individual's quality of life if this course of action is pursued. The individual and his or her family should come to the same conclusions regarding futility as the physician if effective communication is employed. With full understanding of the risks of one last chemotherapy treatment, new comfort care options should be offered. When framed correctly, the individual and his or her family should feel heard and supported by the alternatives presented.

COMMUNICATION, COMPASSION, AND MEDICAL FUTILITY

Communication and compassion are two of the most essential skills necessary when addressing medical futility. The dying individual and his or her family must feel they are cared about, valued, and respected. Often, medical futility is disputed because of feelings of abandonment, perceived lack of humanity, financial and resource issues, and/or an anxiety-driven attempt to avoid the inevitable. Additional influencing factors should also be identified through the use of active listening and effective communication. Often the terminally ill person and his or her family undergo one last struggle to avoid death. Unresolved issues may prevent a willingness to accept this inescapable outcome. Families may want to compensate for past perceived wrongs, or an uninvolved family member may now want to make a show of control, or reconciliation. The underlying cause of conflicts in care opinions can often be discovered with effective communication and redirecting to only consider what is in the best interest of the individual and not the family member.

In the final hours of care, the brother of a 40-year-old gentleman dying of heart failure began to panic and insisted his brother be placed on a ventilator to help him breathe. A health care provider sat with the brother and discussed his request. The brother was asked very compassionately what he hoped to achieve at this point by placing his brother on a ventilator. The brother stated that he thought it would make him more comfortable and maybe buy him some time. The fact that the ventilator would not stop the dying process but could actually prolong it was discussed. Time was taken to explain the changes in breathing that can occur with the dying process and that his brother would not be suffering. The agonal-like breathing that can occur was the way the body shuts down as it prepares to die. The brother began to cry and was comforted by the health care provider as she held his hand and sat with him. The brother finally admitted that he was having a hard time letting go.

Often, conflicts on medical futility can be resolved if basic physiology is provided, concern over the likelihood of increased suffering is expressed, and the loss of quality of life is conveyed in an empathetic, understanding way that demonstrates respect for the dying and their families. Strong communication skills are essential and it is necessary to take the time to help the individual and family accept comfort care over a treatment or procedure that will ultimately just prolong the dying process.

Society must believe the determination of medical futility is an ethical, honest, and compassionate assessment based on the desire to act in the best interest of the individual. It is not based on a need for power, control, financial issues, or limited resources. The identification of medical futility is a challenging one and not taken lightly by medical providers. It is based in compassion and its full understanding is contingent upon effective communication. It is essential to reframe explanations of care to reflect continuing attention and respect and to diminish the sense that needed care is being withheld. Any perception of abandonment should be addressed and a focus on quality should be emphasized.

CHAPTER 4

Establishing Care of the Dying as an Acute Event

The intentional use of an acronym format for the CARES tool was utilized to encourage parallels to be drawn to other respected acronym-based acute care treatment formats. An association with programs such as the American Heart Association's Advanced Cardiac Life Support (ACLS) and Basic Cardiac Life Support (BCLS) was desired to help emphasize the importance of the CARES tool content and to increase respect for the unique skills required to effectively care for the dying and their families.

Care of the dying may not require the same level of technical expertise required in ACLS, but the unique communication and associated supportive skills more than qualify care of the dying as an acute event (Byock, 2012; Quill, 1996). To paraphrase Dr. Timothy Quill, care of the dying may not be high tech; but it is definitely high touch and deserving of treatment as an acute event. The communication and high touch skills required for quality end-of-life (EOL) care require an emphasis in compassion, empathy, and acceptance of individual grieving processes and needs.

HEALTH CARE SYSTEMS AND CARE OF THE DYING

The health care systems in our country have not evolved much in terms of caring for the dying. As Lynn, Lynch Schuster, Wilkinson, and Noyes Simon (2008) noted in their book, *Improving Care for the End of Life*, the lack of attention given to improve care of the dying was overshadowed by numerous gains in medical technology that were providing cures, addressing emergencies, and improving surgery. The many variables involved in a terminal illness could not be fully anticipated and resources continued to focus on curing, not on comfort, as thousands of dying individuals continued to receive inadequate care, and suffer and die in pain. Death was considered a failure of medical management, so it was rationalized that if curative strategies were improved, there would be fewer deaths. Improving upon the dying process seemed futile as the individual was going to die no matter what was provided, so our Western medical culture continued to address death through avoidance.

When improving the dying process was approached, ethical concerns regarding physician-assisted suicide, euthanasia, and the acceleration of the dying process became topics of concern. Often, the dying in a hospital setting would suffer in pain before their death to confirm that the health care provider did not have a role in the dying process. Families were forced to watch their loved ones die suffering and abandoned.

This approach was acceptable until the baby boomers started attaining the age of 65. Now the possibility of death is becoming a concern for 88.5 million adults in the United States who will reach an age of 65 years or older by 2050 (American Medical Association, 2012; Whitbourne & Whitbourne, 2011). Some of these individuals are in positions of political power and are aware of the kind of death that is possible through hospice and have condemned the current lack of care provided to the dying in a hospital setting. This awareness resulted in studies to confirm the poor status of care provided to the dying and prompted the development of palliative care programs.

Over time, simple compassion also played a role in altering the care of the dying. Common sense began to prevail but staffing and resource issues would continue to delay change. This perspective was again reassessed as the population continued to age, and research found that 85% of all deaths in the United States occurred within this 65+ age group. Sixty percent of this group would die in a hospital, and 80% to 90% of their deaths would be expected (Byock, 1997; Thurston, Wilson, & Hewitt, 2011). Changes in care of the dying were again refueled by this age group. Hospice programs increased, and palliative care programs were developed in hospitals throughout the country. The Joint Commission on Accreditation of Healthcare Organizations (JCAHO) now sponsors a hospital palliative care certification that many feel is just a prelude to mandatory palliative care services for all hospitals in the United States.

CARE FOR THE DYING IN A HOSPITAL SETTING

A change in the delivery of care for the dying in a hospital setting is urgently needed. Baby boomers want an active role in decisions about their care, and to have their wishes respected. To meet the demand for improved care of the dying, health care providers must become educated and experienced in providing compassionate, effective evidence-based care. Yet, the average amount of time expended on EOL care education in medical and nursing programs remains 15 hours (Dickinson, 2007). Health care providers continue to express anxiety and difficulty in effectively addressing the needs of the dying, and consider their basic education on care of the dying to be inadequate. Currently practicing health care providers often do not possess any EOL training (Mutto, Cantoni, Rabhansi, & Villar, 2011; Sanchez-Reilly & Ross, 2012).

Research identified common symptom management needs for 80% of the dying to include dyspnea, pain, and/or restlessness/agitation (Walling, Ettner, Barry, Yamamoto, & Wenger, 2011). Family members of the dying often experience acute stress and anxiety as they witness the death of a loved one; and nurses are experiencing moral distress, compassion fatigue, anxiety, and burnout with their attempts to meet the extensive needs of the dying and the family without appropriate education, training, or resources (Parish et al., 2006; Peterson et al., 2010).

The need to recognize the specialized skill set required to effectively care for the dying and their family is reflected in the CARES tool. Like similar treatment-based protocols, the CARES tool is intended to focus on providing evidence-based care options to reduce if not eliminate the suffering that can occur in the dying process.

TREATING CARE FOR THE DYING INDIVIDUAL AS AN ACUTE EVENT

Use of the CARES tool varies from other acronym-based protocols like ACLS in that initiation does not need to wait until there is a crisis. The nurse caring for the dying individual can request medications and treatment changes recommended in the tool be made available and implement if needed. Many of the suggestions in the CARES tool are within the nurses' scope of practice and do not require an order from a physician. Ideally, death should be anticipated, well supported, loving, and peaceful. You cannot make a similar statement about the code that usually accompanies the implementation of ACLS.

The final hours to moments of the dying should be supported by the presence of the nurse caring for them and their families. It is an acute event of a more loving and spiritual nature and hopefully the chaos of running to get supplies, obtaining additional orders, adjusting medications, and calling for emergent treatments is avoided. Technical skills required at this time are the use of touch, a soft and gentle voice, presence, empathy, and demonstration of our humanity. The family members of the dying individual desperately need the caring of the nurse for the dying individual to reassure and confirm that all possible care is being provided. Families need to know that their loved ones are not suffering and the nurse needs to educate them on how to differentiate between suffering and a normal dying process.

These specialized skills to compassionately educate, comfort, and manage final symptom needs of the dying are what the CARES tool tries to emphasize. To adequately provide this evidence-based care, nurses must be available and cannot be pulled away to care for another individual or to assist with some other need on their unit. The final moments of an individual's life should be honored, and if labeling it an acute event allows the nurse to obtain help to assist with the care needed by others assigned to him or her, obtain additional support staff such as chaplains and social workers, and allow nursing assistants to reprioritize their duties to allow them to bring coffee or water to the family then, yes, dying should be considered an acute event.

Staffing adjustments will have the greatest impact when identifying the dying process as an acute event. Historically, staffing did not allow for the kind of one-to-one care advocated by the CARES tool. This has not changed, but it is possible if the staff on a unit agree that care of a dying individual should be considered an acute event and they are willing to devise a plan to meet the staffing challenge. Another nurse could agree or be assigned to monitor any additional person assigned to the nurse caring for the dying individual, nursing assistants could prioritize their duties to include providing food and beverages for the family, other nursing staff could make a point of checking to see if any additional assistance is needed, and unit secretaries can reorganize themselves to assist the family with phone calls and making final arrangements.

Considering the death of an individual an acute event allows for a shift in priorities, and close collaboration of staff to ensure that quality care is provided. This low-tech, high-touch acute event is worthy of the same respect and staff support that is given to any other emergency (Quill, 1996).

Nurses once felt that the needs of the dying and their families were nonexistent or of no importance. Additional assignments were accepted. Nurses were called away, busy with providing care to other individuals they were assigned to, or simply felt they were not needed. The result was an individual dying in a back room hopefully with some family, but in many cases alone, and forgotten until a nurse came to assess and found he or she had died.

This is such a poor testament to nurses whose very core principles include compassion, empathy, and caring holistically for the individuals under their care. Providing quality care for the dying should not differ from any other care nurses provide. Heath care providers' humanity causes them to question how we care for our dying and their families. Their needs may often be greater than the technical care many nurses are trained to provide. Nurses often hesitate to care for the dying because they are made aware of their own mortality, or wish to avoid the grieving and sadness of the families. Many nurses feel they have nothing to offer and feel foolish not providing any "valuable" treatment or medication. They feel they must "do" when in reality they only need to "be." Nurses need to be present, be active listeners, be compassionate, and most of all be genuine and empathetic.

NURSING'S IMPACT ON COMPASSIONATE CARE FOR THE DYING

Many individuals became nurses because they wanted to help and make a difference. What greater difference can a nurse make than to support another human being to die peacefully surrounded by the love of his or her family? Nurses can make a huge difference to the family of the deceased as they take with them a sense of peace knowing everything was done to make their loved one comfortable, that he or she did not suffer, and died peacefully with dignity and surrounded by loving persons. These memories and feelings the family will take home will help them through their grieving and will influence how they manage future losses in their lives. The family may not remember exactly what the nurse did, but they will remember that the nurse cared and honored their loved one. Talk about making a difference!

Caring for the dying individual and their families is a calling and may not be possible for some nurses with their own personal issues. To treat the final hours to moments as an acute event requires the nurse to act as a strong advocate for the dying and their families. There are many ways to support this process and being the primary nurse caring for individuals and their families is not the only way. A nurse who is uncomfortable caring directly for the dying can assist the primary nurse by covering the care of his or her other assignments, helping the family make phone calls, obtain physician's orders as directed, offer coffee, extra pillows, and so on to the family; and contact palliative care team members as requested.

The need to be genuine, open, and comfortable when caring for the dying is paramount and cannot be forced. Many of the skills necessary for caring for the dying can be learned, but if a nurse cannot work comfortably with this specific population his or her responsibility must shift to finding another nurse who can. All focus needs to be on the dying and their families; a nurse can help in other supportive ways as previously discussed. It is important to be honest with yourself.

Use of the CARES tool encourages nurses to be advocates and to work as a team with other nurses on their unit. Increasing knowledge and understanding of the needs of the dying can promote support from additional health care providers. Their awareness of the many tasks required and their willingness to become involved are necessary to elevate care of the dying to an acute event.

This chapter now explores how the principles presented in CARES impacted the care of the example case of Steven and his family first discussed in the introduction of this book.

STEVEN'S STORY

Steven was actively dying from a graft-versus-host disease (GVHD) process that had attacked his lungs. Nurses on the unit readily accepted his dying as an acute event as they came together to support the nurse providing primary care. One nurse offered to monitor the other individual assigned to Steven's primary care nurse, another nurse offered to contact the social worker and chaplain to assist the family, and the unit secretary made arrangements for coffee and juice to be brought to Steven's room for the family.

The nurses on the unit struggled not to overidentify with Steven because he was a nursing student and was the same age as many of them. The nursing unit's atmosphere was a combination of sadness and determination. The only question for the remaining nursing staff was to ask what else they could be doing for Steven.

The following orders were obtained based on the CARES tool prompts in anticipation of their use as Steven continued to decline:

1. Glycopyrrolate 0.4 mg IV every 2 hours as needed for increased oral secretions
2. Oral suctioning prn, instruct and allow family to suction if desired
3. Discontinue isolation precautions
4. Titrate morphine IV infusion for restlessness or agitation
5. Discontinue all further blood draws
6. Discontinue oxygen saturation monitor and alarms
7. Take blood pressures once a shift
8. Turn only if the family requests, and keep head of the bed elevated for comfort

Steven's mother had expressed a desire to be involved in her son's care, and asked if she could suction her son. Oral suctioning is ineffective for secretion control in the dying and often will cause an increase in secretion production, but Steven's mother wanted to feel useful. This is an early example of how care of the dying can quickly shift to the family. Risks versus benefits were weighed and helping the mother feel useful outweighed the minor increase in secretions the suctioning would cause.

Approval was obtained to discontinue the protective isolation so the parents did not need to be gowned and gloved and could have direct contact with their son. This is another example of how care of the dying can shift focus to the family.

Orders were obtained to titrate up the morphine drip for any signs of restlessness or agitation. The pump was currently at 5 mg/hr. The risks versus the benefits of titrating up the morphine drip and causing a further decline in Steven's respirations were reviewed with Steven's parents. They felt they were the best to assess if Steven was having increased pain and viewed a decline in respiration as an inevitable part of the dying process. The parents wanted to decide if the morphine needed to be increased. Their request was honored as the nurse was aware of the loss of control the parents were experiencing and her desire to keep them involved in Steven's care choices. The parents' primary goal was to not let their son suffer.

Procedures and tests were discontinued in an effort to minimize interruptions that would take time away from the parents to be with their son. Blood draws and oxygen saturation monitor and alarms were discontinued.

GUIDING PRINCIPLES FOR THE DISCONTINUATION OF PROCEDURES AND TESTS

A guiding principle for the discontinuation of procedures and tests planned for the dying is to evaluate what would be done with the information once it is obtained. If the goals of care are comfort only and the family has expressed the desire to stop further transfusions, not to provide life-prolonging emergency drugs, and not to advance oxygen support then blood pressures need only be taken once a shift if this is hospital policy, and Steven should only be turned if the family requests. Nurses and other ancillary health care staff need to be aware of the precious time they are taking away from the family of a dying person when they interfere with routine procedures like turning and bathing. Priorities must be acknowledged and the use of compassion and humanity should dictate the care provided an actively dying individual. Too often nurses feel they must remain task focused to be useful when the more compassionate act would be to defer to the family's wishes and minimize unnecessary interruptions.

As professionals the question must be asked, who are we taking care of? In situations of routines, exceptions should be made for the dying. One of the requirements of an advocate is to act in the best interest of the individual you are caring for and his or her family.

The primary care RN remained with the parents and Steven and once she confirmed the parents wanted some privacy she then frequently checked on them and let them know she was available if they needed anything.

Steven's status was reviewed with the charge nurse and a plan was developed not to assign another individual to the care of that primary nurse. All staff were in agreement and they remained focused on supporting Steven, his family, and the primary nurse caring for them.

REFERENCES

American Medical Association. (2012). *The EPEC (Education in Palliative and End-of-Life Care) project*. Retrieved from http://www.epec.net

Byock, I. (1997). *Dying well: Peace and possibilities at the end of life*. New York, NY: Riverhead Books.

Byock, I. (2012). *The best care possible: A physician's quest to transform care through end of life*. New York, NY: Avery.

Dickinson, G. (2007). End-of-life and palliative care issues in medical and nursing schools in the United States. *Death Studies, 31*(8), 713–726.

Lynn, J., Lynch Schuster, J., Wilkinson, A., & Noyes Simon, L. (2008). *Improving care for the end of life: A sourcebook for health care managers and clinicians* (2nd ed.). New York, NY: Oxford University Press.

Mutto, E. M., Cantoni, M. N., Rabhansi, M. M., & Villar, M. J. (2011). A perspective of end-of-life education in undergraduate medical and nursing students in Buenos Aires, Argentina. *Journal of Palliative Medicine, 15*(1), 93–98.

Parish, K., Glaetzer, K., Grbich, C., Hammond, L., Hegarty, M., & McHugh, A. (2006). Dying for attention: Palliative care in the acute setting. *Australian Journal of Advanced Nursing, 24*(2), 21–25.

Peterson, J., Johnson, M., Halvorsen, B., Apmann, L., Chang, P-C., Kershek, S., Pincon, D. (2010). What is so stressful about caring for a dying patient? A qualitative study of nurses' experiences. *International Journal of Palliative Nursing, 16*(4), 181–187.

Quill, T. E. (1996). *A midwife through the dying process: Stories of healing & hard choices at the end of life*. Baltimore, MD: Johns Hopkins University Press.

Sanchez-Reilly, S., & Ross, J. S. (2012). Hospice and palliative medicine: Curriculum evaluation and learner assessment in medical education. *Journal of Palliative Medicine, 15*(1), 116–122.

Thurston, A. J., Wilson, D. M., & Hewitt, J. A. (2011). Current end-of-life care needs and care practices in acute care hospitals. *Nursing Research and Practice*, Article ID 869302, http://dx.doi.org/10.1155/2011/869302

Walling, A., Ettner, S. L., Barry, T., Yamamoto, M. C., & Wenger, N. S. (2011). Missed opportunities: Use of end-of-life symptom management order protocol among inpatients dying expected deaths. *Journal of Palliative Medicine, 14*(4), 407–412.

Whitbourne, S. K., & Whitbourne, S. (2011). *Adult development and aging: Biopsychosocial perspectives* (4th ed.). Hoboken, NJ: John Wiley & Sons.

CHAPTER 5

Identifying the Most Common Symptom Management and End-of-Life Needs of the Dying

A literature review was utilized to explore current evidence-based care of the dying focusing on common symptom management needs. The literature review identified 80% of the dying would develop pain, dyspnea, and delirium as part of their dying process (Andershed, 2006; Becker et al., 2007). Additional concerns for spiritual care and caregiver self-care emerged to confirm that a holistic approach was needed to effectively care for the dying.

Articles for the literature review were included if they were in English, peer reviewed, contained research-based symptom management needs of the dying, and provided study results/conclusions generalizable to a hospital setting. Articles were excluded if they did not focus on symptom management of the actively dying, addressed care issues for the dying not typical of a hospital setting, or were letters to the editors.

Studies in the literature review were selected based on the presence of one or more of the previously listed inclusion criteria and the absence of any exclusion criteria. Of the 5,611 citations obtained, 1,000 were randomly selected based on initial search of title/abstract, 92 potentially relevant studies were identified. All 92 titles and abstracts were accessed and independently reviewed by the author. The intense review resulted in the elimination of 24 studies: 12 did not contain specific symptom management, 8 were not generalizable to the hospital setting, and 4 did not focus on the dying. The detailed review resulted in the identification of 68 articles to be considered for further inquiry. Of the 68 studies, 28 addressed physical symptom management of the dying, 25 focused on spiritual

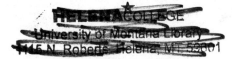

and emotional needs of the dying, and 15 examined health care provider self-care.

The initial literature review suggested that evidence-based end-of-life (EOL) care must include physical symptom management, a spiritual and emotional support focus, and a support system for the health care provider. These preliminary findings are reflected in the organization of the CARES tool. All 68 evidence-based references were reviewed in depth to establish a common focus or symptom management issue for the dying.

Limitations of this study review involve the heavily relied upon use of a clear and detailed abstract, the acceptance of review articles, and articles providing author interpretation or educated opinions on research studies. If the abstract was inadequate, then an important study could be overlooked and potentially limit the findings and conclusions of this review. If the author was biased or overly influenced by psychosocial, cultural, or religious beliefs, then a more conservative focus could be presented not reflective of the general population.

Data collection on care of the dying is made challenging because direct interaction with the dying and their family is rarely ethical. Grieving and a right to privacy greatly limit direct data collection from involved parties. The predominantly descriptive physiologic-based studies used in the review provided standard examples of qualitative research. The review of retrospective data in the form of chart reviews, interviews, and questionnaires supplied the primary source for data. Interviews were confined to health care personnel to avoid any emotional difficulties for grieving families.

The characteristics of the studies were analyzed using numerical frequency and percentages. The chief characteristics of the qualitative exploratory studies included the following: 60% had three to six authors per study; 63% of the studies were written between 2006 and 2013; and all studies were obtained from journals retrieved from electronic databases, were nonexperimental, nursing focused, and conducted in a clinic or hospital setting. Sampling was primarily purposive (90%) with 10% snowball sampling. Data collection was 40% self-report structured interview, 40% self-report focus group or questionnaire, and 20% unstructured participant observation. Only 40% of the studies supplied age ranges of their sample groups; the majority (60%) were listed as adults or elderly adults. Ninety percent of the studies utilized male/female sampling, 20% reported ethnicity, and only 20% utilized nursing or nonnursing theories to guide their research.

Seventy percent of the research studies employed the use of interviews both individual and focused, confirming three core physical symptom management needs of pain (86%), dyspnea (78%), and delirium (60%). Other less frequently cited physical symptom management issues included nausea and vomiting (25%); anxiety (7%); depression (10%); and dysphagia, decubitus formation, diarrhea, fatigue, fever, and myoclonus (3%). The CARES tool did not address any physical symptom management need that occurred less than 60% in the literature review.

PAIN: THE SYMPTOM OF GREATEST CONCERN

Pain continued to be the symptom of greatest concern for the terminally ill during the dying process (Duffy, Payne, & Timmins, 2011; Luhrs et al., 2005). Individuals are continuing to suffer and die in pain because of health care providers' fear and lack of knowledge in pain management for the dying (Brajtman, 2005; Quill, 1996; Radha Krishna, Poulose, & Goh, 2012). An estimated 80% of the dying experience suboptimally treated dyspnea and terminal delirium before death (Del Fabbro, Dalal, & Bruera, 2006; Ellershaw & Wilkinson, 2011). The dismal statistics can be attributed to the discomfort ordering clinicians have for the use of opioids, barbiturates, antipsychotics, and sedatives during the dying process (Byock, 2012; Li, Yeh, Huang, Wang, & Su, 2010).

Knowledge deficits, misconceptions, and unfounded beliefs continue to result in barriers affecting pain and symptom management for the dying (Goodnough, 2013; LeGrand & Walsh, 2011; Radha Krishna, Poulose, & Goh, 2012). The fear of causing harm is counterproductive for the dying and often results in undertreatment and further suffering (Hall, Schroderr, & Weaver, 2002; Henkelman & Dalinis, 1998). Literature has confirmed there is no limit to opioid sedation. It can be titrated to whatever dosage is required to relieve an individual's pain and to maintain desired respiratory status (Bookbinder & Romer, 2002; Constantini, Ottonelli, Canavacci, Pellegrini, & Beccaro, 2011; LeGrand & Walsh, 2011).

Concepts of intent and double effect can greatly assist in guiding humane and ethical symptom management concerns but are often poorly understood (LeGrand & Walsh, 2011; Quill, 1998). The intent or desired outcome of pain and symptom management is to relieve suffering, not to provide euthanasia (Byock, 2012; Quill, 1996). Double effect can be defined as a decision to utilize an intervention with potential side effects or harm when it is determined the benefits outweigh the risks, and the health care provider's intent is to relieve suffering (Kamal, Maguire, Weeler, Currow, & Abernathy, 2012; Quill, 1998). If an actively dying individual writhing in pain is given a bolus of morphine and dies a few moments later, then his or her death can be attributed as much to the disease process as to the opioid (Byock, 2012; Walling, Brown-Saltzman, Barry, Quan, & Wenger, 2008). The double effect was the benefit of reliving an individual's pain. It outweighed the risk of causing death to occur a few moments sooner. Relieving pain and eliminating suffering are the intent and should be the focus of EOL care (Walling et al., 2010).

DYSPNEA

The use of opiates and sedatives to manage dyspnea at EOL also remains complicated by knowledge deficits and personal attitudes often resulting in the denial of dignified comfort measures for the dying (Giovanni, 2012; Hall, Schroderr, & Weaver, 2002). Morphine still remains the gold standard for the prevention of the sensation of suffocation commonly occurring in the terminally ill with advancing respiratory failure (Del Fabbro, Dalal, & Bruera, 2006; Li, Yeh, Huang, Wang, & Su, 2010; Quill, 1998). Quill (1996) noted that suffocation could be one of the most frightening and devastating symptoms the dying must endure; yet physicians and nurses still remain hesitant to provide sedatives and opioids. The concepts of double effect and intent also contribute to the hesitancy of aggressively treating dyspnea (Del Fabbro et al., 2006). The intent is to relieve the sensation of dyspnea and suffocation, not to hasten death. Del Fabbro et al. found that physicians routinely discounted the presence of dyspnea, feeling it was too subjective when not reflected in oxygenation saturations or without the presence of tachypnea. Like pain, dyspnea is a personal perception and should be believed. It can have a basis in anxiety and will often respond to antianxiety agents and distraction, but should never be ignored or dismissed as unreal.

The simple use of a fan was often dismissed as ineffective regardless of research confirmation. A gentle breeze from a fan positioned to blow across the side of the face will stimulate receptors along the trigeminal nerve distribution of the face causing a reduction in perceived dyspnea intensity to be interpreted by the brain (Del Fabbro et al., 2006).

DELIRIUM

Brajtman (2005) cited a 25% to 85% incidence of terminal or restless delirium in the dying. This restless or terminal delirium evolves as a progressive change in cognition, attention, and consciousness over hours (Duffy, Payne, & Timmins, 2011; Hall et al., 2002; Reinke et al., 2010). The symptoms of terminal delirium include restlessness, agitation, confusion, nightmares, and hallucinations. Sedation with antipsychotics and barbiturates is often necessary (Brajtman, 2005; Walling, Ettner, Barry, Yamamoto, & Wenger, 2011). Uncontrolled pain particularly in the elderly can cause confusion and florid delirium. Effective pain management can actually maintain mental clarity (Byock, 2012; Hall et al., 2002). The antianxiety agents lorazepam and midazolam and the antipsychotic agents chlorpromazine and haloperidol are the most frequently used agents cited in literature for the management of terminal and restless delirium (Bookbinder & Romer, 2002; Brajtman, 2005; Del Fabbro et al., 2006).

Some forms of delirium can be resistant to standard medical management and escalate to the point when deeper sedation may be required. This is a very frustrating time for family, as the need for increased sedation may further limit any final communication with the dying (Brajtman, 2005; Constantini et al., 2011). Families are frightened and confused, as agitated or terminal delirium can present as a change in personality and behavior. Effective communication and reassurance from nursing and medical staff will assist the family with acceptance of final cognitive changes (Del Fabbro et al., 2006).

SPIRITUAL AND EMOTIONAL SUPPORT

Spiritual and emotional support was also identified as important EOL care needs in the 68 article literature review. Thirty-five unique themes for nurturing individuals and their family's spiritual needs were identified. Religious expression and rituals comprised 6% ($n = 2$) of the identified needs (see Exhibit 5.1).

EXHIBIT 5.1 Spiritual needs of the dying.

Have a home-like environment	Develop resilience
Feel connected	Transcend fears
Support for family	Be informed
Have privacy	Be reassured
Maintain sense of worthiness	Promote sense of well-being
Maintain dignity	Self-esteem
Be respected	Be treated compassionately
Be listened to	Feel valued
Help to find meaning	Sustain hope
Relief from suffering	Need for holistic support
Treat patient and family as one	Assist with personal anguish
Be treated with empathy	Relief from spiritual pain
Fear of helplessness	Establish care goals
Maintain quality of life	Promote acceptance
Reduce the fear of death and dying	Support religious beliefs and practice
Reduce bereavement-related distress	No fear of becoming burden
Maintain control	No fear of afterlife
Reduce fears of pain, isolation, and the unknown	

The desire to transcend fears of suffering equated with dying was the overall theme for spiritual and emotional support and could encompass 94% (*n* = 33) of the desired assistance requested by individuals and families. The ultimate goal of spiritual and emotional support is to assist the dying and their families to transcend their fears and sufferings and achieve a peaceful death. Transcendence requires supportive actions on the part of the health care provider to promote a sense of connectiveness, preparation, reassurance, dignity, respect, worthiness, well-being, value, strong self-esteem, reduction of fears of an afterlife, dying, pain, and isolation (Boston, Bruce, & Schreiber, 2011; Reinke et al., 2010). Actions to provide identified spiritual needs can be achieved with strong communication skills, active listening, supportive presence, compassion, empathy, and caregiver humanity. Just being present and genuinely listening demonstrates respect and compassion, and may be all that a patient and family need to feel supported and valued (Puchalski & Ferrell, 2010).

Spirituality is essential to the holistic health of patients, their families, and care providers (Hutchinson, 2011). It addresses the "inner reality of human beings" and provides a deeper understanding of life's purpose (p. 151). It is more than religious beliefs and is evident in the values and ethics of all individuals (Dezutter et al., 2009). Spirituality has an important role in patient care and impacts patient belief systems, meaning of life, and concerns about an afterlife (Rubinstein, Black, Doyle, Moss, & Moss, 2011; Taylor, 2002; Wink & Scott, 2005). It is influenced by culture, religion, personal life philosophy; and it can be equated with one's very soul (Coward & Reed, 1996).

Puchalski and Ferrell (2010) defined spirituality as "the aspect of humanity that refers to the way individuals seek and express meaning and purpose, and the way they experience their connectedness to the moment, to self, to others, to nature and to the significant" (p. 16).

Pamela Reed's *Theory of Self-Transcendence* provided the theoretical framework for the CARES tool and is reinforced in the findings of the literature review. Self-transcendence was the desired spiritual and emotional focus and is strongly based in the need for health care providers to support spirituality. To transcend fears and suffering equated with dying, there must be an inner sense of being valued, worthy, and deserving of peace (Edmondson, Park, Chaudoir, & Wortmann, 2008; Kotter-Grühn, Kleinspehn-Ammerlahn, Gerstorf, & Smith, 2009). An individual must feel that his or her life has meaning and he or she is part of a greater purpose (Cobb, Puchalski, & Rumbold, 2012; Kotter-Grühn et al., 2009). The greatest tool a health care provider can possess to nurture a dying person's spirituality is his or her humanity (Emanuel, Alpert, & Emanuel, 2001; Lloyd-Williams, Kennedy, Sixsmith, & Sixsmith, 2007).

Lundberg, Olsson, and Fürst (2013) identified the sense of security and comfort family members obtained from health care providers who took time to clearly explain issues common in the dying process. Families felt prepared and supported as they experienced grief and loss. The health care provider's interactions were simple open caring demonstrations of concern, but families felt they drew inner strength and courage from the encounters. Patients and their families need to be treated as one unit, and they are deserving of the health care provider's attention and support (Hui, Thorney, Delgado-Guay, & Bruera, 2011). Empathy and compassion are essential and will help minimize the risk of psychological trauma for the family as they attempt to endure their grief and sense of loss (Delgado-Guay et al., 2011; Moss, 2001; Wright et al., 2010).

As families experience grief and loss, they are also attempting to adapt to life without their loved one. Such feelings often produce a magnified sense of vulnerability and abandonment. These feelings can be tempered, if not totally eliminated, by a health care provider who takes the time to just be present, to actively listen, and to demonstrate compassion and understanding through touch or assistance with personal requests (Downey, Curtis, Lafferty, Herting, & Engelberg, 2010).

Dying alters how an individual is perceived and implies new expectations for family members. Pamela Reed (1987) noted that it is at this vulnerable time that self-transcendence can occur if individuals and/or their family's fears and anxieties are tempered by having their spiritual needs met. Families and patients need to feel valued, possess dignity, and be respected (Edmondson et al., 2008; Hui et al., 2011; Nilmanat et al., 2010; Tamura et al., 2005). Spiritual needs can often be addressed by simply providing a cool washcloth for a patient's forehead or an extra chair or blanket for the family. The action is minimal, but the associated underlying statement implies the health care provider respects the needs of the individual and wants to make him or her feel comforted, cared for, and valued (Hayden, 2010; McClain-Jacobson et al., 2004; Nazarko, 2012).

Additional supportive behaviors by health care providers were identified by Williams, Lewis, Burgio, and Goode (2012) as behavioral competencies supplied by the American Association of Colleges of Nursing (AACN) in their publication, *A Peaceful Death: Recommended Competencies and Curricular Guidelines for End-of-Life Nursing Care*. The additional supportive behaviors include assisting with coping, suffering, grief, loss, and bereavement; communicating effectively and compassionately; treating patients holistically; and respecting a patient's views and wishes.

Moss (2001) further clarified necessary supportive behaviors for the health care provider by identifying five domains of quality EOL care that were important to patients as:

1. Receiving adequate pain and symptom management

2. Avoiding inappropriate prolongation of dying

3. Achieving a sense of control

4. Relieving burden on loved ones

5. Strengthening relationships with loved ones (p. 149)

The addition of spiritual and emotional care to evidence-based symptom management allows total patient and family care. This complete physical and psychosocial care is essential to providing quality EOL care and to confront any associated holistic suffering (Boston et al., 2011; Jacobsen, Holland, & Steensma, 2012).

SELF-CARE FOR THE HEALTH CARE PROVIDER

Suffering can also be experienced by the health care provider. The final focus of the literature review was the identification of the need for health care provider self-care. Twenty-two percent of the review articles cited this important need. It encompasses not only the professional nurse, but also included anyone providing direct care for the terminally ill.

Caring for the dying and their family can be very stressful (Kearney, Weininger, Vachon, Harrison, & Mount, 2009; Murray-Frommelt, 1991). There are often multiple demands for time, and tasks rarely are completed as thoroughly as desired (Peterson et al., 2010; Sinclair, 2011). Many ethical dilemmas can arise as medical personnel adjust to the stress of caring for the actively dying.

Moral distress develops as personal core values and perceptions of care perceived as essential are ignored or somehow rendered unrealistic due to staffing, resources, or the absence of administrative support (Lange, Thom, & Kline, 2008; Mutto, Errazquin, Rabhansi, & Villar, 2010; Peterson et al., 2010). Issues of unjustifiable life support and unnecessary tests and treatments continue to provide the greatest source of moral distress for medical and nursing staff as they struggle in the role of patient advocate (Parish et al., 2006; Sinclair, 2011).

Psychological distress can develop in the presence of moral distress and manifest as loss of self-worth, anxiety, depression, helplessness, dread, anguish, and compromised integrity (Leung et al., 2011; Wakefield, 2000). Ong, Yee, and Lee (2012) noted a direct relationship between emotional exhaustion and burnout. Self-care is essential when working in high-stress areas such as emergency rooms, intensive care units, and areas providing care for the actively dying.

A common challenge for health care providers caring for the dying is overidentification as staff recognize similar life circumstances and family issues (Braun, Gordon, & Uziely, 2010; Rhodes-Kropf, Meier, & Adelman, 2003; Sinclair, 2011). Overidentification can result in further compassion fatigue, patient and family avoidance, and distancing if the caregiver remains unaware of his or her faulty coping mechanisms and does not utilize self-care options (Murray-Frommelt, 1991; Parish et al., 2006; Sinclair, 2011).

The literature review noted 15 articles emphasizing self-care. They identified 54 issues that could impact a health care provider's emotional health, such as stress, a sense of failure, the need for meaning, and a loss of purpose. The issues could be consolidated into three major areas of focus to promote self-care: (a) the need for self-awareness, (b) experience, and (c) education.

Self-care must incorporate self-awareness of the impact a caregiver's own culture, life experiences, attitudes, and fears have on the care he or she is providing. There must be a separation of personal bias and negative issues about death to allow supportive, focused, compassionate, and empathic EOL care. Much of the development of self-awareness occurs with the remaining two areas of focus: (a) the need for education and (b) the need for experience.

Evidence-based education on care of the dying can provide the health care provider an understanding of professional grieving and professional boundaries, how to provide holistic care, addressing one's own bias, understanding and reframing one's sense of failure, knowing how to seek validation, identifying meaning, and embracing the importance of the work one does for the dying and their families.

Nurses continue to have the greatest contact with the dying and remain the primary decision makers for titration and obtaining necessary medications and orders to provide compassionate care for patients. Their role as a patient advocate is essential. With this important role comes the responsibility to ensure that all components necessary to provide a peaceful death are in place to support a dying patient and family in his or her final journey (Jack, Gambles, Murphy, & Ellershaw, 2003). This responsibility was identified as highly stressful in the literature review for nurses as palliative care is a reflection of nursing values and philosophy they often must struggle to achieve (McHugh, Arnold, & Buschman, 2012). Through self-awareness, education, and experience, nurses can reduce their stress levels and provide quality evidence-based care for the dying.

Experience provides practice and acceptance of the knowledge gained from care of the dying. Comfort with communicating, maintaining a supportive presence, and actively listening evolves only with practice. Experience can emphasize the importance of small kindnesses and supporting the patient and family holistically.

Self-care encourages reflection and allows for the recognition of positive outcomes. Open discussion and review of cases and personal reflections on professional role and ability can promote self-awareness, stimulate sharing of information, provide additional education, and assist others with developing methods to work more effectively with the dying. A rediscovering of priorities, spirituality, meaning, life purpose, and reduced anxiety about death are often reported with the use of individualized self-care activities (Frommelt, 2003; McHugh et al., 2012; Schwartz et al., 2005).

The compassionate and caring attitude that freely allows people to display their humanity can often permeate interactions with coworkers and within personal lives. A satisfaction of knowing one made a difference in the lives of a dying patient's family is often very rewarding and sustains many health care providers in their long careers of caring for the dying (Byock, 2012; Puchalski & Ferrell, 2010).

Self-care activities also include taking vacations, enjoying hobbies, and participating in activities that can relax and recharge the health care provider. EOL health care providers must become experts on self-care (Sinclair, 2011).

REFERENCES

Andershed, B. (2006). Relatives in end-of-life care-part I: A systematic review of the literature the last five years, January 1999–February 2004. *Journal of Clinical Nursing, 15*, 1158–1169.

Becker, G., Sarhatlic, R., Olschewski, M., Xander, C., Momm, F., & Blum, H. E. (2007). End-of-life care in hospital: Current practice and potentials for improvement. *Journal of Pain and Symptom Management, 33*(6), 711–719.

Bookbinder, M., & Romer, A. L. (2002). Raising the standard of care for imminently dying patients using quality improvement. *Journal of Palliative Medicine, 5*(4), 635–644.

Boston, P., Bruce, A., & Schreiber, R. (2011). Existential suffering in the palliative care setting: An integrated literature review. *Journal of Pain and Symptom Management, 41*, 604–618.

Brajtman, S. (2005). Helping the family through the experience of terminal restlessness. *Journal of Hospice and Palliative Nursing, 7*(2), 73–81.

Braun, M., Gordon, D., & Uziely, B. (2010). Associations between oncology nurses' attitudes toward death and caring for dying patients. *Oncology Nursing Forum, 37*(1), 43–49.

Byock, I. (2012). *The best care possible: A physician's quest to transform care through end of life.* New York, NY: Avery.

Cobb, M., Puchalski, C. M., & Rumbold, B. (Eds.). (2012). *Oxford textbook of spirituality in healthcare.* New York, NY: Oxford University Press.

Constantini, M., Ottonelli, S., Canavacci, L., Pellegrini, F., & Beccaro, M. (2011). The effectiveness of the Liverpool care pathway in improving end-of-life care for dying cancer patients in hospital. A cluster randomized trial. *Biomedical Central Health Services Research, 11*(13).

Coward, D. D., & Reed, P. G. (1996). Self-transcendence: A resource for healing at the end of life. *Issues in Mental Health Nursing, 17*, 275–288.

Del Fabbro, E., Dalal, S., & Bruera, E. (2006). Symptom control in palliative care-Part III: Dyspnea and delirium. *Journal of Palliative Medicine, 9*(2), 422–437.

Delgado-Guay, M., Hui, D., Parsons, H. A., Govan, K., De la Cruz, M., Thorney, S., & Bruera, E. (2011). Spirituality, religiosity, and spiritual pain in advanced cancer patients. *Journal of Pain and Symptom Management, 41*, 986–994.

Dezutter, J., Soenens, B., Luyckx, K., Bruyneel, S., Vansteenkiste, M., Duriez, B., & Hutsebaut, D. (2009). The role of religion in death attitudes: Distinguishing between religious belief and style of processing religious contents. *Death Studies, 33*, 73–92.

Downey, L., Curtis, J. R., Lafferty, W. E., Herting, J. R., & Engelberg, A. (2010). The quality of dying and death (QODD) questionnaire: Empirical domains and theoretical perspectives. *Journal of Pain and Symptom Management, 39*(1), 1–15.

Duffy, A., Payne, S., & Timmins, F. (2011). The Liverpool care pathway: Does it improve quality of dying? *British Journal of Nursing, 20*(15), 942–946.

Edmondson, D., Park, C. L., Chaudoir, S. R., & Wortmann, J. H. (2008). Death without God: Religious struggle, death concerns, and depression in the terminally ill. *Psychological Science, 19*, 754–758.

Ellershaw, J., & Wilkinson, S. (2011). *Care of the dying: A pathway to excellence* (2nd ed.). New York, NY: Oxford University Press.

Emanuel, L. L., Alpert, H. R., & Emanuel, E. E. (2001). Concise screening questions for clinical assessments of terminal care: The needs near the end-of-life care screening tool. *Journal of Palliative Medicine, 4*, 465–474.

Frommelt, K. H. (2003). Attitudes toward care of the terminally ill: An educational intervention. *American Journal of Hospice and Palliative Medicine, 20*(1), 13–22.

Giovanni, L. A. (2012). End-of-life care in the United States: Current reality and future promise—A policy review. *Nursing Economics, 30*(3), 127–135.

Goodnough, A. (2013, January 10). *As a nurse lay dying, offering herself as instruction in caring.* South Hadley, MA: The New York Times.

Hall, P., Schroderr, C., & Weaver, L. (2002). The last 48 hours of life in long term care: A focused chart audit. *Journal of the American Geriatrics Society, 50*(3), 501–506.

Hayden, D. (2010). Spirituality in end-of-life care. *British Journal of Community Nursing, 16*, 546–551.

Henkelman, W. J., & Dalinis, P. M. (1998). A protocol for palliative care measures. *Nursing Management, 29*(1), 40–46.

Hui, D., Thorrney, S., Delgado-Guay, M., & Bruera, E. (2011). The frequency and correlates of spiritual distress among patients with advanced cancer admitted to an acute palliative care unit. *American Journal of Hospice and Palliative Medicine, 28*(4), 264–270.

Hutchinson, T. A. (2011). *Whole person care: A new paradigm for the 21st century.* New York, NY: Springer Publishing.

Jack, B. A., Gambles, M., Murphy, D., & Ellershaw, J. E. (2003). Nurses' perceptions of the Liverpool Care Pathway for the dying patient in the acute hospital setting. *International Journal of Palliative Nursing, 9,* 375–381.

Jacobsen, P. B., Holland, J. C., & Steensma, D. P. (2012). Caring for the whole patient: The science of psychosocial care. *Journal of Clinical Psychology, 30,* 1151–1186.

Kamal, A. H., Maguire, J. M., Weeler, J. L., Currow, D. C., & Abernathy, A. P. (2012). Dyspnea review for palliative care professional: Treatment goals and therapeutic options. *Journal of Palliative Medicine, 15*(1), 106–114.

Kearney, M. K., Weininger, R. B., Vachon, M. L. S., Harrison, R. L., & Mount, B. M. (2009). Self-care of physicians caring for patients at the end-of-life. *Journal of American Medical Association, 301,* 1155–1164.

Kotter-Grühn, D., Kleinspehn-Ammerlahn, A., Gerstorf, D., & Smith, J. (2009). Self-perceptions of aging predict mortality and change with approaching death: 16-year longitudinal results from the Berlin aging study. *Psychology and Aging, 24,* 654–667.

Lange, M., Thom, B., & Kline, N. E. (2008). Assessing nurses' attitudes toward death and caring for dying patients in a comprehensive cancer center. *Oncology Nursing Forum, 35,* 955–959.

LeGrand, S. B., & Walsh, D. (2011). Comfort measures: Practical care of the dying cancer patient. *American Journal of Hospice and Palliative Medicine, 27,* 488–493.

Leung, D., Esplen, J., Peter, E., Howell, D., Rodin, G., & Fitch, M. (2011). How haematological cancer nurses experience the threat of patients' mortality. *Journal of Advanced Nursing, 68,* 2175–2184.

Li, M.-H., Yeh, E.-T., Huang, S. C., Wang, H.-M., & Su, W.-R. (2010). Clinical experience with strong opioids in pain control of terminally ill cancer patients in palliative care settings in Taiwan. *Journal of Experimental and Clinical Medicine, 2*(6), 292–296.

Lloyd-Williams, M., Kennedy, V., Sixsmith, A., & Sixsmith, J. (2007). The end of life: A qualitative study of the perceptions of people over age 80 on issues surrounding death and dying. *Journal of Pain and Symptom Management, 34*(1), 60–66.

Luhrs, C. A., Meghani, S., Homel, P., Drayton, M., O'Toole, E., Paccione, M., & Bookbinder, M. (2005). Pilot of a pathway to improve the care of imminently dying oncology inpatients in a veterans affairs medical center. *Journal of Pain and Symptom Management, 29*(6), 544–551.

Lundberg, T., Olsson, M., & Fürst, C. J. (2013). The perspectives of bereaved family members on their experiences of support in palliative care. *International Journal of Palliative Nursing, 19*(6), 282–288.

McClain-Jacobson, C., Rosenfeld, B., Kosinski, A., Pessin, H., Cimino, J. E., & Breitbart, W. (2004). Belief in an afterlife, spiritual well-being and end-of-life despair in patients with advanced cancer. *General Hospital Psychiatry, 26*, 484–486.

McHugh, M. E., Arnold, J., & Buschman, P. R. (2012). Nurses leading the response to the crisis of palliative care for vulnerable populations. *Nursing Economics, 30*(3), 140–147.

Moss, A. H. (2001). Measuring the quality of dying. *Journal of Palliative Medicine, 4*, 149–152.

Murray-Frommelt, K. H. (1991). The effects of death education on nurses' attitudes toward caring for terminally ill persons and their families. *American Journal of Hospice and Palliative Medicine, 8*(5), 37–43.

Mutto, E. M., Errazquin, A., Rabhansi, M. M., & Villar, M. J. (2010). Nursing education: The experience, attitudes, and impact of caring for dying patients by undergraduate Argentinian nursing students. *Journal of Palliative Medicine, 13*, 1445–1450.

Nazarko, L. (2012). Aspirations of immortality. *British Journal of Community Nursing, 17*(5), 205–206.

Nilmanat, K., Chailungka, P., Phungrassami, T., Promnoi, C., Tulathamkit, K., Noo-urai, P., & Phattaranavig, S. (2010). Living with suffering as voiced by Thai patients with terminal advanced cancer. *International Journal of Palliative Nursing, 16*, 393–399.

Ong, W., Yee, C. M., & Lee, A. (2012). Ethical dilemmas in the care of cancer patients near the end of life. *Singapore Medical Journal, 53*(1), 11–14.

Parish, K., Glaetzer, K., Grbich, C., Hammond, L., Hegarty, M., & McHugh, A. (2006). Dying for attention: Palliative care in the acute setting. *Australian Journal of Advanced Nursing, 24*(2), 21–25.

Peterson, J., Johnson, M., Halvorsen, B., Apmann, L., Chang, P.-C., Kershek, & S., Pincon, D. (2010). What is so stressful about caring for a dying patient? A qualitative study of nurses' experiences. *International Journal of Palliative Nursing, 16*(4), 181–187.

Puchalski, C. M., & Ferrell, B. R. (2010). *Making health care whole: Integrating spirituality into patient care*. West Conshohocken, PA: Templeton Press.

Quill, T. E. (1996). *A midwife through the dying process: Stories of healing & hard choices at the end of life*. Baltimore, MD: Johns Hopkins University Press.

Quill, T. E. (1998). Principal of double effect and end-of-life pain management: additional myths and a limited role. *Journal of Palliative Medicine, 1*(4), 333–336.

Radha Krishna, L. K., Poulose, V. J., & Goh, C. (2012). The use of midazolam and haloperidol in cancer patients at the end of life. *Singapore Medical Journal, 53*(1), 62–66.

Reed, P. G. (1987). Spirituality and well-being in terminally ill hospitalized adults. *Research in Nursing & Health, 10*, 335–344.

Reinke, L. F., Shannon, S. E., Engelberg, R., Dotolo, D., Silvestri, G. A., & Curtis, J. R. (2010). Nurses' identification of important yet under-utilized end-of-life care skills for patients with life-limiting or terminal illness. *Journal of Palliative Medicine, 13,* 753–759.

Rhodes-Kropf, J., Meier, D., & Adelman, R. (2003). Interns learning to care for dying patients. *Journal of Palliative Medicine, 6,* 865–872.

Rubinstein, R. L., Black, H. K., Doyle, P. J., Moss, M., & Moss, S. Z. (2011). Faith and end of life in nursing homes. *Journal of Aging Research,* vol. 2011, Article ID 390427, 1–7. doi: 104061/2011/390427

Schwartz, C. E., Clive, D. M., Mazor, K. M., Ma, Y., Reed, G., & Clay, M. (2005). Detecting attitudinal changes about death and dying as a result of end-of-life care curricula for medical undergraduates. *Journal of Palliative Medicine, 8,* 975–987.

Sinclair, S. (2011). Impact of death and dying on the personal lives and practices of palliative and hospice care professionals. *Canadian Medical Association Journal, 183*(2), 180–187.

Tamura, K., Ichihara, K., Maetaki, E., Takayama, K., Tanisawa, K., & Ikenaga, M. (2005). Development of a spiritual pain assessment sheet for terminal cancer patients: Targeting terminal cancer patients admitted to palliative care units in Japan. *Palliative and Supportive Care, 4,* 179–188.

Taylor, E. J. (2002). *Spiritual care: Nursing theory, research, and practice.* Upper Saddle River, NJ: Prentice Hall.

Wakefield, A. (2000). Nurses' response to death and dying: A need for relentless self-care. *International Journal of Palliative Care Nursing, 5*(6), 245–251.

Walling, A., Asch, S. M., Lorenz, K. A., Roth, C. P., Barry, T., Kahn, K. L, & Wenger, N. (2010). The quality of care provided to hospitalized patients at the end of life. *Arch International Medicine, 170*(12), 1–13.

Walling, A., Brown-Saltzman, K., Barry, T., Quan, R. J., & Wenger, N. S. (2008). Assessment of implementation of an order protocol for end-of-life symptom management. *Journal of Palliative Medicine, 11,* 857–865.

Walling, A., Ettner, S. L., Barry, T., Yamamoto, M. C., & Wenger, N. S. (2011). Missed opportunities: Use of end-of-life symptom management order protocol among inpatients dying expected deaths. *Journal of Palliative Medicine, 14,* 407–412.

Williams, B. R., Lewis, D. R., Burgio, K. L., & Goode, P. S. (2012). Next-of-kin's perceptions of how hospital nursing staff support family presence before, during, and after the death of a loved one. *Journal of Hospice and Palliative Nursing, 14,* 541–550.

Wink, P., & Scott, J. (2005). Does religiousness buffer against the fear of death and dying in late adulthood? Findings from a longitudinal study. *Psychological Sciences, 60B*(4), 207–214.

Wright, A. A., Keating, N. L., Balboni, T. A., Matulonis, U. A., Block, S. D., & Prigerson, H. G. (2010). Place of death: Correlations with quality of life of patients with cancer and predictors of bereaved caregivers' mental health. *Journal of Clinical Oncology,* 1–8.

PART II

The CARES Tool

CHAPTER 6

CARES Tool: Organization and Considerations

The CARES tool, in addition to assisting nurses with delivery of evidence-based care of the dying and viewing the care of the dying as an acute event, also needed to be portable and readily accessible. The volumes of research and reference materials available on care of the dying were condensed to include the most common symptom management needs. An extensive review of the literature found the most basic common needs of the dying included pain management and comfort measures, breathing assistance, control of delirium, emotional and spiritual support, and self-care for caregivers.

The following issues and concerns helped organize and shape the final version of the CARES tool and are discussed in detail.

1. Nurses receive little to no education on care of the dying.

2. Nurses feel they have minimal time to attend in-services, and can be resistant to learning new skills.

3. The uneducated nurse can feel abandoned and helpless when caring for the dying.

4. Communication is the foundation for end-of-life care, it does not come naturally and reminders are necessary to prompt important conversations.

5. Nurses need to know what care they can provide within their scope of practice.

6. Nurses will be caring for more dying patients because of our aging population; and 80% to 90% of the deaths will be expected.

7. The final hours to moments of a dying patient's life can be very stressful for the nurse. The CARES tool's suggestions and prompts can have a calming effect and assist the nurse in remaining focused.

8. The skills required for the care of the dying directly mirror those required to be an effective and compassionate nurse in any situation.

9. Access to basic principles involved in caring for the dying can be helpful when there is an immediate symptom management need.

10. The nurses' past personal and professional experiences with death can greatly impact the care they provide dying patients and their families.

LITTLE TO NO EDUCATION ON CARE OF THE DYING

Dickinson (2007) estimated an average of only 15 hours was dedicated to education on the care of the dying. Some palliative care experts feel this estimation is generous and interject their concern over the education deficiencies that exist within the current nursing workforce. Educational programs are available through associations such as the National Board of Certification for Hospice and Palliative Nursing (NBCHPN), the Association for Death Education and Bereavement Counseling (ADEC), the American Association of Colleges of Nursing (AACN) and their End-of-Life Nursing Education Consortium (ELNEC) program, and the physician-focused Education in Palliative and End-of-Life Care (EPEC) program.

Independent learning is essential. There is a wealth of information available on care of the dying, and the desire to develop his or her skills must drive the individual's initiative to self-educate. Extensive information is available online, in published educational references, and through peer-reviewed articles. There are numerous websites with quality information and associations such as the Coalition for Compassionate Care, Compassion and Choice, AARP, and additional sites to explore under key phrases such as end-of-life care, care of the dying, palliative care, and hospice. Learning must be made a priority by the nurse and certification through the NBCHPN is encouraged and available with an advanced, general, or administrative nursing focus.

Universities and nursing education programs are progressively adding education on care of the dying into their curriculum, but a significant void still exists and can only be corrected with individual dedication to learning and the desire to network with others possessing similar interests. Taking the ELNEC program is a good place to start. Further information on this program can be obtained through the AACN website, www.aacn.nche.edu/ELNEC.

MINIMAL TIME TO LEARN NEW SKILLS

The hospital-based nurse providing bedside care often finds it difficult to attend lectures and in-services at their own facility. They are even more challenged when asked to attend off-campus seminars. Staffing issues are a common reason for the inability to attend continuing education sessions. More typical is the low priority nurses places on education, given their many personal priorities regarding family and home care needs.

An improved level of importance can occur when adult learning principles are addressed. Nurses must feel there is an urgency or recognize a need to learn a new skill. Often, a new skill is mandated by management. Mandating an adult to accomplish a task often results in the learning of the technical skills or motions required to complete the task, but there is often no buy-in or recognition of importance that will make the new skill a welcomed and utilized addition to the nurses' skill set.

If nurses have a sense of urgency to learn a new skill they will make more of an effort to arrange their schedule to attend a course. Utilizing learning opportunities online is a more convenient option to consider as discussed earlier. Ultimately it is the nurse that must make his or her learning a priority.

Nurses are more likely to make learning a priority if they are:

- Involved in actively identifying the need to learn more about caring for the dying
- Allowed to provide input into the development or application of a newly identified skill set
- Supported and provided resources to successfully develop a new skill set
- Encouraged to become invested in the goal of improving care for the dying through mentoring, education, and by example
- Instilled with a passion to improve their care of the dying by educators that emphasize the strategic role nurses have as advocates for promoting a peaceful death
- Given credit for the personal and professional knowledge and abilities they already possess, and shown how they can adapt this knowledge into a new skill set

Nurses must be open, compassionate, and empathetic. These behaviors are essential and, like any new skill, they must be practiced so that they become standard responses. The families of dying patients are hypersensitive and can identify forced, stiff, and unnatural behavior. They will have a tendency not to call a nurse exhibiting behaviors that imply discomfort or uncertainty because of fears they may anger, cause inconvenience, or annoy them. Opportunities to promote a peaceful death can be lost.

The CARES tool can help a nurse be more comfortable when caring for the dying as it emphasizes the need to be open and genuine. The tool attempts to address evidence-based common symptom management needs, emotional and spiritual needs and issues, and reminds the health care provider to explore any personal baggage that may impact his or her care. It is intended to address the holistic needs of the patient and family and to identify the supportive needs of the health care providers. The CARES tool is designed to promote self-transcendence for all parties involved in the dying process and to encourage the important use of our humanity.

FEELINGS OF ABANDONMENT AND HELPLESSNESS

The sensation of feeling abandoned exists for both the nurse caring for a dying patient and the family of a dying patient. Perceptions of abandonment can occur on several levels. For nurses, abandonment issues may be centered on:

- The lack of assistance offered by coworkers because they believe caring for a dying patient is simple and does not require any additional help
- The feeling they have no emotional outlet for feelings related to care of the dying because they may be perceived as unprofessional
- Orders for basic symptom management needs of the dying may be difficult to obtain because physicians tend to avoid these patient requests or fail to return pages because they deem order requests for a dying patient a low priority
- Lack of awareness of the emotional, spiritual, and psychological support available through assigned social workers and chaplains, and through requesting a palliative care consults; nurses do not need to be the sole support for dying patients and their families
- Hesitation over requesting help from other nursing staff because of the fear of being viewed as incompetent, inexperienced, overemotional, and/or unorganized

Families of dying patients often develop a sense of abandonment because:

- Their loved ones are in the process of dying, leaving them at least physically for the rest of their lives.
- Their lives will be forever changed because of this death. They may be forced to abandon their dreams for education, travel, and personal identity in an effort to fill the void created by the death of their loved one.
- Nurses will often avoid entering the dying patient's room because they perceive there is nothing to do or out of discomfort being near a dying patient. Rather than feel awkward because they are uncertain of what to

do to comfort the families of the dying, nurses will commonly avoid any interactions.

The CARES tool acknowledges the feelings of abandonment and provides suggestions and prompts in the sections on emotional and spiritual support and self-care. Both sections emphasize the need for communication, compassion, and to seek out resources of support. Nurses need to accept they are human and professional grieving is an acceptable practice. The CARES tool prompts are not intended to be fulfilled just by the individual health care provider. Nurses are encouraged to utilize their resources and to acknowledge that no one individual is ever expected to function in isolation. Just as other coworkers should seek out opportunities to assist with the care of a dying patient not under their direct supervision, it is also the responsibility of the nurse providing care to ask for help and guidance. Often as human beings, we are primarily accountable for our feelings of isolation and need to take the initiative to resolve them.

APPROPRIATE COMMUNICATION SKILLS

Communication is the very foundation of compassionate, empathetic, and evidence-based care of the dying. It is addressed in detail in Chapter 15. The focus of caring for the dying is on identifying and supporting the needs of the individuals and their families, the use of therapeutic listening and presence, the support of hope, celebrating the individual, and separating him or her from the disease. Communication is based on empathy, promoting transcendence, and utilizing our humanity. The dying have no choice over the course of their lives, but they do have a choice on how they spend their remaining time. Through communication their goals of care can be honored, they can have loving peaceful closure time with their family, and they can die peacefully. It is all possible with therapeutic, open, honest, and compassionate communication.

SCOPE OF PRACTICE

The CARES tool encourages nurses to seek patient and family involvement in care decisions. This is encouraged through communication, active listening, and the nurse acting as an advocate for their needs. So much of the disease and dying process is out of the patient and family control. Any opportunity to regain some control by allowing them to make any decision, no matter how small, can be comforting. The tool suggests that patients and families be given the right to decide if they want labs drawn, tube feedings, monitors, blood pressures, and scheduled turning to be provided. The dying and their family should be the guardians of what precious time remains for closure and a life without each other.

Many if not all of the actions do not require an order from a physician. They are common issues that require the nurse to act as a patient advocate. Acknowledging and supporting the goals of care, as the patient and their family defined them, is one example requiring the advocacy role. The CARES tool tries to encourage nurses to embrace their responsibility to deliver quality evidence-based care to this extremely vulnerable patient population.

AN INCREASING AGING POPULATION

In 2014, 78 million adults turned 68 years old (Becker et al., 2007). By 2050, it is predicted there will be more persons on this planet age 65 and over than individuals age 15 and younger. This age shift has never before occurred in human history. We are all becoming painfully aware of the staggering increases that will continue to occur with our aging populations, and the effects they will have on our health care resources.

Health care providers must improve their knowledge and delivery of geriatric and palliative care, and become experts in the care of the dying. There remains a massive void between the education currently provided to nurses and the escalating needs of the patient population they will serve. The CARES tool was designed to assist in this education and to provide a reference for nurses to address the most common symptom management needs of the dying they will encounter.

EXPECTED HOSPITAL DEATHS

Research has shown 80% to 90% of all deaths that occur within a hospital setting are expected. This finding reinforces the need to explore if goals of care are being obtained for these individuals, if hospital resources are being fully utilized, and ultimately, if nurses are adequately trained to address this important patient population's needs.

The fact that the majority of deaths in a hospital is anticipated further emphasizes the education and training needs for nurses. There is an ongoing need to improve communication skills, to obtain and maintain pain and airway management skills, and to improve and consistently utilize treatments for delirium and emotional and spiritual distress.

The CARES tool provides needed information nurses will require to obtain medication orders, stimulate necessary conversations, and address commonly occurring symptom management needs. Further education to fully understand the needs of the dying is continually encouraged.

STRESS IN THE FINAL HOURS TO MOMENTS
OF THE DYING PROCESS

The CARES tool provides a focus for the nurse during the often chaotic final hours to moments of the dying process. The easy to recall acronym can act as a list for the nurse to inventory as he or she inevitably struggles with the question "have I done everything I can?" This question can often trouble a nurse after a death as nagging self-doubt clouds the review of his or her care.

Nurses are taught to fix and death goes against all of our training. Death is unavoidable for all of us. It should be viewed as a natural process of living. When a nurse begins to question their skills, the self-doubt can be devastating. This self-doubt can be compounded in the final moments of care. The CARES tool can take the emotional doubt out of the moment and allow for nurses to reassess and organize their thoughts as they review the sections of the tool. This emotional break can help to diffuse the anxiety and sadness that can occur during the final moments of life for a family and for the nurse. The distraction can be very helpful.

The CARES tool section on self-care is an essential part of the tool. It addresses the emotional impact that caring for the dying can have on the nurse or health care provider. It reminds us all that we are human, we will have an emotional response to death, and we will often need an outlet to work through our personal and professional feelings. Again, communication is paramount. Nurses must verbalize their needs, accept that they have a right to seek emotional and spiritual comfort, and realize that having an emotional response to death is not a sign of weakness or incompetence.

SKILLS REQUIRED FOR CARE OF THE DYING

The CARES tool encourages nurses to seek the dying individual and the family's involvement in care decisions. This is encouraged through communication, active listening, and the nurse acting as an advocate for their needs. So much of the disease and dying process is out of the individual and family's control. Any opportunity to regain some control by allowing them to make any decision, no matter how small, can be comforting. The tool suggests that dying and their families be given the right to decide if they want labs drawn, tube feedings, monitors, blood pressures, and scheduled turning to occur. The dying and their families should be the guardians of what precious time remains for closure and a life without each other.

The specific skills required for care of the dying are not high tech, they are high touch (Quill, 1996). It is the ability to convey to dying individuals and their families that they are respected, valued, and deserving of your care. Communication skills are essential as compassion, empathy, and genuine kindness must be second nature in the effort to assist with the achievement of a peaceful death.

Understanding methods to control common symptoms that occur during the dying process are important such as knowing how to manage pain, prevent the anxiety of dyspnea and fear of suffocating, and how to regulate or minimize delirium.

Nurses must be actively present, therapeutic listeners, and have a grasp of basic physiology to explain in lay terms the differences between a normal dying process and suffering. The CARES tool can assist with prompts that suggest the need for certain skills in specific situations. The best preparation for developing skills for care of the dying is through education from formalized conferences, courses, and through independent study.

IMMEDIATELY ADDRESSING SYMPTOM MANAGEMENT NEEDS

The CARES tool was intended to be a very basic summary of the important symptom management needs commonly encountered by the dying and their families. It best functions as a brief reminder of the extensive literature now available, and can help the nurse to quickly identify orders they should request and conversations to anticipate. It is not intended to be a substitute for the learning that can only be obtained from such programs as ELNEC, or other formal care of the dying courses. The CARES tool is a "CliffNote" version of the in-depth research-based information available on care of the dying. It is a quick reference tool to prompt nurses and help them remember the more in-depth teaching they have hopefully been given. The CARES tool is intended to stimulate the reader to seek a more detailed understanding of the unique needs and skills required to effectively care for this much underserved patient population.

IMPACT OF NURSES' PAST PERSONAL AND PROFESSIONAL EXPERIENCES

One of the greatest challenges of caring for the dying is the influence of the personal baggage we carry. Even the most professional nurse cannot help but be influenced by past suffering he or she has personally and professionally witnessed, and will either retreat in fear of experiencing the same emotional pain and trauma or be resolved to prevent the same events from reoccurring.

Nurses must become aware of the baggage they carry and commit to possible resolutions, such as:

- Professional counseling, attend grief and bereavement support groups, work with spiritual counselors

- A transfer to other areas of nursing where death is not common or a part of the patient care population
- Making a conscious choice to gain experience and arrange to work with a preceptor or coworker more comfortable with caring for the dying
- Asking coworkers to take over their assignment when personal and professional situations are too overwhelming
- Accepting assignments to care for the dying knowing additional support persons are available to assist you if needed such as social workers, chaplains, experienced coworkers, and psychologists; and recognizing only through experience and education will a nurse ever become skilled caring for the dying
- Accepting that no one is a natural at caring for the dying, and care can never be fully accomplished in isolation, that skills must be learned, experience gained, and individuals who can act as resources must be identified and utilized to provide quality evidence-based care for the dying

There is an amazing bonus that can occur when caring for the dying: nurses can actually become more whole. Often this occurs even when nurses are not aware that any aspect of their life was broken. Nurses can learn real compassion, they are a witness to true love and courage, and they begin to learn what is really important in life. Many nurses experienced in caring for the dying view their work as a privilege and are humbled by the opportunity they are given to care for the dying.

Whenever a nurse has the ability to make a difference and provide compassion and support for a dying individual and his or her family, similar negatively perceived events the nurse may have encountered in personal or professional experiences will begin to heal. Learning about care of the dying can continue this healing process. Nurses can often dismiss and forgive the many issues they may have carried with them that contributed to what they identified as past failures. Education and experience can provide perspective and assist in the identification of the unavoidable. Both can play an integral role toward learning about the many components necessary to promoting a peaceful death and reduce the anxiety associated with second guessing treatment decisions. Knowledge and the ability to apply it with compassion while preserving the dignity and value of the dying are self-healing experiences. Just knowing the difference you made in the lives of a grieving family because of your efforts can also be a rejuvenating experience and add to self-healing.

The suggested reading section in Chapter 25 can provide extensive educational resources and individualized learning about care of the dying. Learning effective evidence-based skills and providing them to the dying and their families are both appreciated by the recipients and allow for personal growth and healing for the nurse.

There are few opportunities in life that can provide as much positive reinforcement for why you became a nurse as when you care for the dying and their families. The CARES tool was developed to allow nurses to experience the gift that can occur when you are invited to assist a fellow human being on his or her final journey in this life.

This gift is only possible if the nurse can be emotionally open and has the ability to embrace the vast knowledge to be gained. The CARES tool provides a beginning and is intended to encourage learning. When we learn to effectively and compassionately care for the dying it will change our lives. We will have the potential to help families through their grieving process and to grow as human beings.

REFERENCES

Becker, G., Sarhatlic, R., Olschewski, M., Xander, C., Momm, F., & Blum, H. E. (2007). End-of-life care in hospital: Current practice and potentials for improvement. *Journal of Pain and Symptom Management, 33,* 711–719.

Dickinson, G. (2007). End-of-life and palliative care issues in medical and nursing schools in the United States. *Death Studies, 31,* 713–726.

Quill, T. E. (1996). *A midwife through the dying process: Stories of healing & hard choices at the end of life.* Baltimore, MD: Johns Hopkins University Press.

CHAPTER 7

Comfort

The CARES tool addresses the broad subject of comfort by focusing on the physical needs of the dying. Emphasis is directed toward effective pain management and eliminating unnecessary interruptions between the dying and their families. The comfort section of the CARES tool attempts to encourage creating as much time as possible for the family to create final loving memories and obtain some measure of closure.

There are two parts to the comfort section of the CARES tool. The first focuses on pain management, and the second provides prompts and suggestions to eliminate interruptions to the grieving process for the dying and their families. The comfort section promotes the discontinuation of unnecessary procedures, medications, treatments, and monitoring. This can be accomplished by nurses effectively communicating rationale based on changes that occur within the body during the dying process and decisions not to treat abnormal test results and allow a natural death to occur. It is essential that nurses phrase the suggestion to discontinue blood work, monitors, or procedures in a positive light and not as something to be taken away. Fears of abandonment, inadequate care, and feelings of unworthiness must be dispelled. Nurses need to clearly communicate that the discontinuation of some care is because it unnecessarily interferes with established goals of care, the general comfort of the loved one, and/or precious personal time available for the family.

The comfort section of the CARES tool emphasizes the important role of patient advocate. It encourages nurses to act in the best interest of the individuals under their care through the use of effective communication, anticipation of needs, and the promotion of a peaceful death. A strong patient advocate works to ensure the dying individual's wishes are known and all parties involved are fully informed prior to any decision-making process.

PART I: PAIN MANAGEMENT

Acting as an advocate for pain relief is an essential role of the nurse. Statistics available on the incidence of individuals dying in pain range from 50% to 90% (Byock, 1997; Quill, 1996). Byock (2012) noted there was no excuse for an individual to die in pain given the available resources and current technology of our society, yet, painful deaths continue to occur. Reasons for this discrepancy in providing quality evidence-based pain management are due to the following.

1. **An inability to effectively assess or believe the presence of pain.** The need of the health care provider to believe complaints of pain has proven to be a challenge. If an individual is noted sleeping, breathing at a normal rate (16–18 respirations/min), with warm and dry skin; some caregivers would hesitate to believe they are in pain. Pasero and McCaffery (2011) noted pain to be a subjective experience and should be believed. Many cultures believe in not openly expressing pain. Distractions such as sleep, a hug from a child, or a television program can distract from the pain perception but that does not mean pain does not exist. Alternative pain therapies are based on the brain's inability to focus on two strong stimuli at the same time. Health care providers must be cautious not to pass personal judgment on the existence of pain. Strong pain assessment skills are needed and family interpretations of the dying individual's mannerisms and facial expressions should be taken under consideration.

2. **Limiting opioids or not providing opioids out of fear of causing premature death or being accused of providing euthanasia or physician-assisted suicide.** There are no set limits on opioid dosing for pain management. The dose is titrated to effect. High doses will be necessary for opioid tolerant individuals. Once an opioid level is considered excessive and pain is still not controlled, a change to a different opioid with a slightly different mechanism of action may be helpful. The dying process alters how an opioid is circulated and absorbed and will be unique to every individual. The addition of a benzodiazepine such as Ativan in a continuous infusion may be helpful as anxiety will increase the perception of pain. There is an ethical dilemma that can develop when medicating a dying individual for pain and understanding and finding comfort with the concepts of intent and double effect become crucial. If the intent was to relieve the dying individual's pain and they died moments after receiving an opioid, it does not mean they died of an overdose. It could just as easily mean the individual succumbed to their disease. The concept of double effect occurs when pain medication is given to relieve pain with the knowledge that the patient may die because of the escalating dosage. Again, intent is considered and the

intent was to decrease the dying individual's pain. The Supreme Court established intent as the primary factor to be proven in euthanasia and physician-assisted suicide cases (Quill, 1998). Many health care providers will choose to refrain from further opioid dosing because of the fear of expediting death and opt to let the individual die in pain rather than risk future legal action against them.

3. **The desire to confirm progressing unresponsiveness is the result of the dying process and not overmedication of opioids.** Often health care providers will encounter a change in mental status particularly with the actively dying. This unresponsiveness is often a normal course of the dying process and not a side effect of the opioid, especially in an opioid-tolerant individual. Reducing the opioid may cause the individual to become more alert because their level of pain has increased. The ethical question becomes: Is it reasonable to keep a dying individual in pain just because of the fear of expediting that individual's death? Is not medicating an actively dying individual who is in pain only prolonging his or her dying process, and how is that even remotely humane? An even more profound question becomes who are we, as health care providers, really taking care of? In most cases we are protecting ourselves and continue to allow the dying to suffer and die in pain.

4. **Misunderstandings or lack of knowledge about opioid tolerance and addiction.** Some health care providers set a personal limit on the amount of opioids they will provide an individual and feel exceeding that limit may indicate implied approval or support of the dying individual's addiction. First, the difference between tolerance and addiction must be understood. Individuals on long-term opioid therapy will eventually tolerate the medications and most of the side effects of the drug will resolve except for constipation. This resolution of side effects implies the individual has become "tolerant" of the medication. This tolerance will also result in the need for increased dosing as more opioid will be required to produce the same level of pain relief. The body may have adjusted to more effectively metabolize the medication, and/or pain receptors may require more medication to slow pain stimuli transmission to the brain. There is no psychological attachment, no desire for an escape from feelings, and the pain remains very real to the individual. Addiction typically includes a psychological attachment and a need for ever-increasing amounts of a medication after the physical need has resolved. When a person is dying, our own personal code of ethics must be closely examined. What purpose is served by allowing the dying to suffer? If the dying individual has a tolerance to some opioids or an addiction problem, it now becomes irrelevant. They are dying and their death will soon negate any concerns (Pasero & McCaffery, 2011).

5. **Cultural beliefs, family desire to maintain communication, and religious atonement.** Often, issues specific to family beliefs or customs may impact pain management for the dying. Compassionate listening and communication are required to fully inform the family so decisions on care can be made based on physiology and not just emotion. Families may require gentle redirection of needs to reflect more on what will benefit the dying individual and not just the family member. Is the need to talk to the dying more important than relieving his or her pain? Is the belief that an individual must suffer to be absolved of their sins to enter heaven truly in the best interest of a dying person screaming in pain? Often these issues do not have a compromise, but as a patient advocate the nurse must attempt to question care decisions that are not perceived as being in the best interest of the dying. Family meetings with the health care team and an ethics consult may resolve these issues. Occasionally a court order is needed but, sadly, the time required to obtain one may take longer than the remaining days to hours of the dying individual's life.

Additional teaching points for effective pain management include informing the dying individual and their family how quickly a drug should work and how soon additional medication can be provided. Medications given intravenously reach peak effect in about 15 minutes. Oral medications can take 60 minutes to reach maximum effectiveness. Subcut injections require 30 minutes to become fully effective, and transdermal medications will require 6 to 8 hours.

The use of continuous IV opioids and boluses is another common educational need for a dying person and his or her family. The plan for titration of the continuous infusion should be reviewed and it is essential the nurse be readily available to make needed changes. Teaching on the use of the bolus should include that only the dying person and the nurse can deliver the bolus if this is the agreed upon arrangement.

The need for sustained blood levels of an opioid and the concept of breakthrough pain may require frequent clarification. Again, issues of double effect and intent would still apply. It is important that family members are informed of these ethical issues and verbalize understanding and support. The nurse may need to re-educate the family and provide numerous discussions on the ethics of pain management to ensure the family's comfort.

Even the most compassionate and complete discussions of pain management for the dying may not avoid a family member's discomfort with treatment. Occasional 911 calls have been placed, arguments between family members have erupted, and threats to health care staff have been made. All this acting out can commonly be traced back to unresolved relationship issues with family members and the dying or just the general fear of dying the family member has now personalized. It is important to remember if a family is dysfunctional before a crisis they will typically become even more dysfunctional during a crisis. The nurse and the health care team must continue to act in the best interest of the dying individual. The use of security and the barring of certain family members may be necessary.

Pain management for the dying can be complicated by many issues other than the physical presence of pain. The perception of pain is enhanced by anxiety and fear. It often has psychosocial, cultural, spiritual, and emotional components. The nurse needs to keep the dying person comfortable and calm and the family will typically respond the same way.

Other key points to consider listed in the CARES tool include:

- There is no maximum dose of opioids for pain control.
- There will always be a last dose when caring for a dying patient.
- Keep in mind the legal and ethical concepts of intent.
- The patient is dying because of their disease process and not the opioid.
- Adjustments in dosage or type of opioid may be required in the presence of renal failure.
    a. Consider fentanyl.
    b. Opioids stay in the system longer with renal failure. Dosage is usually smaller.
- Consider changing the type of opiate if pain remains uncontrolled.

PART II: PROMOTING PHYSICAL COMFORT AND INCREASING DIRECT INTERACTIONS WITH THE DYING AND THEIR FAMILIES

The primary focus of care for the dying patient is comfort. This section of the CARES tool addresses what can be done to promote physical comfort and to increase time available for direct interactions between the dying and their families. All unnecessary procedures, tests, and activities should be evaluated as time for the patient and family to be together is now the priority. The nurse, acting as patient and family advocate, should communicate with the family and provide them the option of requesting certain tasks, procedures, and monitoring be stopped or modified. Again, the nurse must phrase these modifications of care and monitoring not as something being taken away, but rather as tasks, procedures, medications, and so on, which can be stopped because they serve no useful purpose, take time away from the family and their loved one, and/or are painful or no longer necessary. The goals of care should be honored and the desire to be kept comfortable and have quality time with family must take precedence over routine and hospital policy.

The CARES tool comfort section, Part II, prompts the nurse to consider obtaining orders as appropriate:

1. **Stop or modify vital signs, turn off monitors and alarms, and stop or decrease labs.** If the dying person is a do not resuscitate (DNR), to stop or decrease the obtaining of vital signs is reasonable. No treatment is planned for this information and its collection only challenges the decision not to treat. Health care providers and family members may waver in their resolve to stop all aggressive management and question if they should attempt one last treatment or procedure. This "second guessing" can result in providing treatment and procedures that only prolong dying. Family and health care providers must keep in mind that treating low blood pressure will not alter the underlying disease, such as cancer or heart disease. It will just take longer for the individual to die, and there is no guarantee that the extra time given will be quality time. The health care provider and the family must acknowledge how the dying individual defines quality. If the dying individual believes that existing on machines or medications and the loss of the ability to care for oneself is not quality, then the nurse acting as the patient's advocate must make the dying person's wishes clear.

2. **Stop oral and all nonessential medications if the patient is unable to swallow.** The inability to swallow occurs in the dying process when energy and stimulation to activate muscle groups is lost. If swallowing becomes difficult, the dying are more likely to choke, obstruct their airway, and/or aspirate. A dying individual can actually die sooner if made to continue oral medications in the presence of dysphagia.

3. **Clarify IV options (stop or reduce).** The continuation of IV fluids often becomes a concern for the family as they do not want their loved one to dehydrate or become thirsty. Family should be reassured that in the normal course of dying, the body no longer senses thirst. The use of IV solutions has proven ineffective in promoting hydration in an actively dying individual. The dying have reduced albumin and colloidal osmotic pressure is lost. They can no longer keep fluid in the vascular space to impact blood pressure. The fluid will migrate into the local tissues and cause increased peripheral edema. IV fluids can be infused at a keep-open rate just to appease the family. Continuing IV fluid at a keep-open rate per family request is often one of the first care issues the nurse will provide for the family's comfort and marks the transition of care focus to the family as the dying become more unresponsive.

4. **Stop or reduce tube feedings.** The issue of whether to stop nourishment is complicated by cultural associations of equating food with love. Fears of having their loved one starve to death must be tempered

by the nurse as he or she shares some basic physical changes occurring in the body of the dying. Some basic rationales to share include:

a. A natural loss of appetite occurs during the dying process to allow for additional blood to be shunted from the gut to the heart, lungs, and brain where it is most needed (Becker et al., 2007).

b. Any food consumed will not be adequately digested and the dying will most commonly vomit and could aspirate (Winter, 2000).

c. Actively dying persons do not experience hunger or thirst (Hallenbeck, 2000).

d. It is extremely difficult for the dying to benefit from food intake due to reduced ability to digest and the fact that the energy needs of the disease will be fed over normal body function (Ferrell & Coyle, 2010; Winter, 2000).

e. The increase in energy expenditure, likelihood of aspiration, and additional pain and suffering that accompany the use of tube feedings in the terminally ill can actually cause them to die sooner (Winter, 2000).

5. **Discontinue isolation.** The need for isolation when caring for the dying should be clarified with a member of the infectious disease department. If isolation is protective it can be easily discontinued. Measures must still be taken to prevent possible transmission of disease to other individuals in the institution. A modified isolation plan can be developed to allow skin contact with the dying as long as effective hand washing is used.

6. **Comfort measures that do not require a physician's order.**

a. Turn and position patient only for comfort and to family request.

b. Modify bathing or stop per family request.

c. Consider reinforcing dressings only.

d. Provide frequent oral care.

e. Provide oral suctioning if family requests. Provide temperature comfort measures such as a cool washcloth and ice packs.

f. Explain that mottling and cyanosis is part of the dying process and not from being cold.

Much of the care provided an actively dying patient should be based on family input. The family can participate in providing these comfort measures if they desire as it also provides them with a sense of involvement.

The ultimate comfort care that can be provided is effective pain management. Pain control for the dying continues to improve with the education of the health care provider, but still remains deficient. The legal and ethical issues associated with pain management continue to complicate this very important aspect of caring for the dying.

STEVEN'S SYMPTOM MANAGEMENT

In an effort to provide use of the CARES tool as it would apply to the sample case of Steven, specific orders and planned care suggested under the comfort section of the CARES tool will be reviewed. Much of the comfort issues were supplied in Chapter 4.

The comfort measures already suggested and discussed included:

1. Discontinuation of protective isolation
2. Titration up of the morphine IV infusion currently at 5 mg an hour for restlessness or agitation at the request of the parents
3. Discontinuation of further blood draws
4. Discontinuation of the oxygen saturation monitor and alarms
5. Reducing the frequency of obtaining blood pressures to once a shift
6. Turning/repositioning only if the family requests, and keeping the head of the bed elevated to comfort

It is essential that stopping procedures or removal of equipment is not viewed by the family as a reduction in care, or an indication that they are being abandoned. Steven's parents were told the goal now was to give them as much uninterrupted time as possible with Steven. Only equipment or treatments no longer contributing to this goal would be stopped. An emphasis on **increasing and adding** to the quality of Steven's care must be emphasized. Nurses must be aware of how they frame their responses to stress, of the importance of family time to allow for closure, and supportive grieving.

The parents' primary goal was to not let their son suffer. The primary care RN remained with the parents and Steven as much as possible, and once she confirmed the parents wanted some privacy began to frequently check on them and let them know she was available if they needed anything.

The daily staffing plan for the unit was amended to allow the primary care nurse time to be available for Steven and his family. The nurses on the unit agreed to cover any new admissions and assisted the primary nurse as requested. All unit staff were in agreement and they remained focused on supporting Steven, his family, and the primary nurse caring for them.

REFERENCES

Becker, G., Sarhatlic, R., Olschewski, M., Xander, C., Momm, F., & Blum, H. E. (2007). End-of-life care in hospital: Current practice and potentials for improvement. *Journal of Pain and Symptom Management*, *33*(6), 711–719.

Byock, I. (1997). *Dying well: Peace and possibilities at the end of life.* New York, NY: Riverhead Books.

Byock, I. (2012). *The best care possible: A physician's quest to transform care through end of life.* New York, NY: Avery.

Ferrell, B. R., & Coyle, N. (Eds.). (2010). *Oxford textbook of palliative nursing* (3rd ed.). New York, NY: Oxford University Press.

Hallenbeck, J. (2000). Fast facts and concepts #10: Tube feed or not tube feed. *Journal of Palliative Medicine, 5*(6), 909–910.

Pasero, C., & McCaffery, M. (2011). *Pain assessment and the pharmacologic management.* St. Louis, MO: Mosby Elsevier.

Quill, T. E. (1996). *A midwife through the dying process: Stories of healing & hard choices at the end of life.* Baltimore, MD: Johns Hopkins University Press.

Quill, T. E. (1998). Principal of double effect and end-of-life pain management: Additional myths and a limited role. *Journal of Palliative Medicine, 1*(4), 333–336.

Winter, S. M. (2000). Terminal nutrition: Framing the debate for the withdrawal of nutritional support in terminally ill patients. *American Journal of Medicine, 109*(9), 723–726.

CHAPTER 8

Airway

The airway section of the CARES tool addresses the dyspnea that occurs during the active dying process for 80% of the population (Hall, Schroderr, & Weaver, 2002; Kamal, Maguire, Weeler, Currow, & Abernathy, 2012). The End-of-Life Nursing Education Consortium (ELNEC) program lecture on symptom management (2013) listed the diseases most commonly associated with dyspnea, which are lung disease, heart disease, stroke, dementia, end-stage renal disease, and metastatic cancer.

Much of the care required to effectively manage dyspnea is centered on education for the family, as they will require assistance to differentiate between the irregular often agonal breathing that occurs during a normal dying process and suffering.

Respiratory failure that progresses while the dying individual is still alert can be one of the most frightening sensations the dying will endure, and the most challenging to manage. The treatment for this sense of suffocating is the use of antipsychotics and/or antianxiety agents, and benzodiazepines to reduce additional oxygen requirements created by increasing anxiety.

OPIOIDS AND SEDATIVES IN THE MANAGEMENT OF DYSPNEA

The use of opiates and sedatives to manage dyspnea at end of life (EOL) is standard medical management. Knowledge deficits and personal attitudes still result in undermedicating and suffering at the EOL. This can only be corrected through further education and experience for nurses and primary caregivers. Lynn, Lynch Schuster, Wilkinson, and Noyes Simon (2008) noted that if a primary caregiver is confident in his or her abilities to manage dyspnea for an actively dying patient he or she is aware of the importance of avoiding any sense of suffocation. Nurses hesitate to increase pain medication because it can cause respiratory arrest. If they watch their patients closely, they can continue to increase pain medication and stop once the patient becomes increasingly sleepy.

The most common medication used for the treatment of dyspnea is morphine. This seems counterintuitive, but the rationale behind the use of morphine involves not just its sedative effects but also its ability to improve coronary circulation thus improving cardiac function and oxygen transport.

The concern over associated respiratory failure with the use of morphine remains a point of apprehension for many health care providers. This is a rare side effect for most dying patients because of opioid tolerance acquired over years of treatment. All patient groups require close monitoring as the respiratory failure associated with opioid overdose occurs after a change in mental status. This greatly diminished responsiveness or hypersomnolence, as discussed earlier, can be quickly identified and measures taken to reverse the effects of the opioids before premature respiratory failure occurs in a dying patient. Alternative methods to reduce respiratory distress in the dying should be considered if oversedation is a concern.

Any method to reduce pain and anxiety can assist in reducing respiratory distress. A calm and supportive environment and use of therapeutic touch by the family and nurse is essential. Another approach to reducing perceptions of shortness of breath encountered during the dying process is the use of a fan at a low setting positioned to gently blow across the side of the patient's face. This gentle stream of air stimulates the trigeminal nerve to lessen the sensation to the brain of air hunger or shortness of breath. A fan can also help circulate the air, making breathing easier. Repositioning to an upright sitting position can allow for fuller expansion of the chest cavity allowing the diaphragm more room to descend. Providing calming music, distractions with television, or being read to can all assist in reducing anxiety and associated dyspnea. The nurse should continue to frequently assess pain status and achieve a balance in medications that both relieves anxiety, pain, and assists the breathing process.

Ultimately, the progressive slowing and irregular breathing patterns that occur during the dying process cannot be solely attributed to pain medications. The individual is dying and respiratory failure is a component of the dying process.

The sedative effects of morphine can help individuals relax and expend less energy resources that can further reduce the workload of the heart. The reduction of stress both physical and psychological can actually result in prolonging life (Ferrell & Coyle, 2010). Regardless of the research evidence confirming the effectiveness of morphine, the use of morphine to treat dyspnea for a dying patient still remains controversial for many practitioners.

TREATMENT OF OROPHARYNGEAL SECRETIONS

The dying process also results in the pooling of oropharyngeal secretions causing loud congestive sounds. Patients can become restless and anxious in the early stages of the dying process if this occurs, but classically oropharyngeal pooling of secretions is more commonly observed with decreased responsiveness and is an ominous sign of death within hours to days. The pooling of oropharyngeal secretions occurs with the loss of muscle strength and control to effectively clear the airway and the inability of functional epithelial cilia to propel secretions downward. Unless an increase in agitation is assessed, this process is rarely uncomfortable for the dying, but can be very disconcerting for their families. The treatment is to provide medication such as glycopyrrolate, scopolamine patch, or atropine 1% ophthalmic solution to reduce the amount of secretion production. These medications are highly effective but can cause excessive mucosal dryness. Aggressive oral care will be needed to counteract this dryness (Freeman, 2013).

Another alternative treatment for pooling oropharyngeal secretions is to provide oral suctioning. This is commonly ineffective as secretions will readily repool and frequent oral suctioning can cause an increase in secretion production, but it provides a task for the family to perform and helps them feel useful. This is an early example of how care of the dying begins to shift its focus to the needs of the family. Providing tasks for the family can help to create some distraction from their grief, help them feel useful, and give them an outlet to demonstrate their love for the dying family member.

ADDITIONAL CONSIDERATIONS

An additional useful task for the family is to encourage them to speak directly to their loved one. Research still confirms the ability to hear exists long after the ability to respond is lost during the dying process. The nurse should emphasize the calming effects of touch and talking using statements of love and reassurance.

The challenge of caring for the dying with respiratory distress and associated anxiety occurs when the individual receiving pain medication and sedation becomes more unresponsive. This "new" or increasing unresponsiveness is also a "classic" characteristic of the dying process and associated respiratory function decline. Opioid overdose is commonly not the underlying cause. It is often difficult to accurately assess the cause of the progressive unresponsiveness. Respirations stop with death, and nurses must be confident in their intent to relieve the patient's suffering and avoid second guessing themselves. Unfortunately, in many cases a decision will be made to reverse the effects of opioids. This can result in the dying individual becoming more alert and aware of his or her pain, struggle to breathe, and forced to die suffering.

The decision to wean down opioids should be weighed against risks versus benefits. Is it ethical and compassionate to reduce sedation for a dying patient so his or her pain response will return and stimulate breathing? The question becomes, who are we treating? Health care providers want to ensure their treatment management does not accelerate the dying process or cause the individual to die prematurely. There is often less concern over causing the individual to die in pain than there is to confirm that death was not a direct cause of opioid overdosing. The fact that the patient is dying from a terminal disease must be taken into the equation when determining the best possible care. Ethically the decision to continue pain medication while an individual is dying falls under the issue of intent. The nurse's intent is to relieve their pain not hasten their death.

Often the irregular and gasp-like breathing commonly seen in a dying individual is a response just prior to dying and is the result of exclusive brain stem innervations and is not voluntary. It is the body's final attempt to pull oxygen into dying tissues. At this point, the patient is unaware of his or her breathing and is no longer responsive. The family may remain concerned over what they interpret as continued struggling to breathe and will require education and much reassurance.

The decline of respirations in the dying process can progress in a variety of patterns involving alternating rapid respirations with episodes of apnea. Ultimately, there is a slowing of the rate of respirations and irregular patterns may become even more irregular. Often there are longer and longer periods of apnea until no respirations are attempted. Again, the slowed irregular breathing patterns that occur with the active dying process cannot be solely attributed to pain medication. The individual is actively dying.

The CARES tool lists suggestions to manage breathing complications and reminds the nurse that the use of supplemental oxygen during the dying process is often ineffective. Dyspnea is very subjective and can be equated with anxiety and pain. ELNEC (2013) noted there is often little correlation between subjective responses and oxygen levels. Providing supplemental oxygen may help to minimize the family's fears of their loved one suffering, but may not provide any physiological support for the dying individual. It is important to review the goals of care established by the patient and family regarding supplemental oxygen, and for the nurse to reassure the family when they voice concerns regarding suffering. It is often necessary to interject during the active stage of dying that the use of supplemental oxygen will not affect the disease process that is causing their loved one to die, in some cases it may only prolong the dying process.

As the family watches their loved one decline, it is common for them to begin to second guess their care decisions because of fears that their loved one is suffering. Changes in breathing can become one of the most upsetting physical changes in the dying process for the family to watch. The nurse must educate the family on the changes that will occur in breathing as part of the dying process and help them differentiate end-stage gasp-like respirations from suffering. Research has shown the irregular agonal respirations often accompanied by accessory muscle involvement are typical responses to exclusively brain stem innervation. Higher level brain function and other systemic respiratory regulating systems are no longer functioning. This ominous physical finding confirms that death will soon occur. Little can be done to reduce the appearance of agonal respirations, repositioning may diminish or lessen some of the associated spastic movements.

The withholding or noninitiation of treatment and the withdrawing or discontinuation of treatment were considered the same by the Supreme Court. No ethical or medical distinction can be made (DeSpelder & Strickland, 2015). This applies to providing supplemental oxygen and withdrawing oxygen support.

The removal of ventilatory life support in terminally ill and dying patients was not specifically addressed in the CARES tool. It can be a very complicated decision for families, and if at all possible should be avoided through effective communication based on risks versus benefits and quality-of-life goals. It should be emphasized the individual will not suffer if not intubated as sedation will be provided and holistic care of their needs will continue.

All the suggested measures for secretion and airway management would apply post extubation. It is recommended individual hospital policy and procedures are followed for terminal extubations and to continue the emphasis on comfort by utilizing antianxiety agents and opioids as directed by the physician.

STEVEN'S SYMPTOM MANAGEMENT

When assisting Steven and his family through the dying process, it was extremely important to help the parents recognize the normal breathing changes that were occurring with Steven's suffering. Steven's respirations were agonal. His emaciated body would spasm and his chest would arch forward with each open-mouthed breath. The BiPAP machine was forcing oxygen into his rigid lungs and only added to the spasm-like response of his respirations. If Steven was uncomfortable it would be from the BiPAP and the family was informed of the need to possibly reduce the volume of oxygen delivered to make Steven more comfortable.

The parents were gently told the BiPAP was just prolonging Steven's dying process and causing him more discomfort. They were aware of how to reduce the settings on the BiPAP machine and requested the machine be turned down. The option to turn the BiPAP off and place Steven on a nasal cannula was introduced and the parents chose to stay with the current treatment plan.

The mother asked if she could suction her son when his oral secretions began to pool at the back of his throat. She expressed concern that the excessive secretions may be making Steven uncomfortable. An oral suction device was provided.

I was aware that suctioning would be ineffective and Steven would continue to have pooling secretions. I was also aware that suctioning would decrease the amount of oxygen being delivered to Steven and could cause him to die sooner.

Steven no longer possessed voluntary reflexes for gag, corneal, or pupillary responses. His death was imminent and suctioning would not alter this course. It was now an opportunity to care for the mother and help her feel she was involved with the care of her son. Suctioning would be a distraction from her grief and a way to demonstrate her love for her son. It was just suctioning, yet it could give this loving mother an opportunity to care for Steven one last time, as she had all his life. It could provide a moment of normalcy that would give her an emotional break from reality and allow her to recall a time when she cared for her son as a child when he would run to her for comfort.

Years later, Steven's mother may not remember the actual act of suctioning, but she will remember the peace and emotional comfort that the act provided. This memory will greatly assist her during the bereavement process as she will find comfort in knowing she did everything she could to comfort her son.

Steven's parents chose to have the BiPAP turned down slowly and to increase the morphine drip if his respirations became more agonal. Steven's body no longer arched with the BiPAP's forced breaths and he appeared to be resting more comfortably even as his mother suctioned his mouth every few minutes and moistened his lips.

REFERENCES

DeSpelder, L. A., & Strickland, A. L. (2015). *The last dance: Encountering death and dying* (10th ed.). New York, NY: McGraw-Hill.

Ferrell, B. R., & Coyle, N. (Eds.). (2010). *Oxford textbook of palliative nursing* (3rd ed.). New York, NY: Oxford University Press.

Freeman, B. (2013). CARES: An acronym organized tool for the care of the dying. *Journal of Hospice and Palliative Nursing, 15*(3), 147–153.

Hall, P., Schroderr, C., & Weaver, L. (2002). The last 48 hours of life in long term care: A focused chart audit. *Journal of the American Geriatrics Society, 50*(3), 501–506.

Kamal, A. H., Maguire, J. M., Weeler, J. L., Currow, D. C., & Abernathy, A. P. (2012). Dyspnea review for palliative care professional: treatment goals and therapeutic options. *Journal of Palliative Medicine, 15*(1), 106–114.

Lynn, J., Lynch Schuster, J., Wilkinson, A., & Noyes Simon, L. (2008). *Improving care for the end of life: A sourcebook for health care managers and clinicians* (2nd ed.). New York, NY: Oxford University Press.

CHAPTER 9

Restlessness and Delirium

Brajtman (2005) cited an incidence of terminal or restless delirium in 25% to 85% of actively dying patients. This neuropsychiatric disorder can be treatable if caused by polypharmacy, infections, bladder distention, fecal impaction, or pain (Close & Long, 2012). Urinary tract infections are one of the most common causes of delirium. The use of antibiotics for an individual who is actively dying should be discussed in an effort to honor established goals of care and to explore the risks versus benefits of potentially prolonging the dying process.

Close and Long (2012) noted risk factors for the development of delirium before an individual begins the active dying process. The risk factors include:

- Advancing age
- Pre-existing cognitive impairment
- Severity of illness
- Depression
- Vision or hearing impairment
- Functional impairment (p. 378)

Other literature resources included additional risk factors such as being male, alcohol abuse, immobilization, dehydration, malnutrition, metabolic abnormalities, and sleep deprivation.

PATHOPHYSIOLOGY OF DELIRIUM

The onset of delirium is acute. This rapid onset is what differentiates delirium from dementia and some encephalopathies. The pathophysiology of delirium is focused on alterations in cerebral oxygenation, altered neurotransmission, plasma esterase activity disturbances, and the production of proinflammatory cytokines. In addition, varied metabolic and ischemic brain insults can also produce delirium. Examples of these pathologic processes include hypoxemia, hypercapnia, hypoglycemia, and major organ dysfunctions. The body's production of proinflammatory cytokines is stimulated with tissue injury that commonly results from infection, trauma, organ failure, and surgery. Elevated serum proinflammatory cytokines in compromised vulnerable individuals can cause severe inflammation of the brain and are directly associated with the development of delirium in susceptible individuals such as the elderly and the dying (Close & Long, 2012).

Ellershaw and Wilkinson (2011) estimated that 50% of all terminal delirium cases have no known etiology. There is a belief that delirium during the dying process is a result of increasing anoxia to the brain. The process results in brain cell death and associated behavioral changes. This is also the time when the dying claim to see previous family members or other individuals who have died. There are many theories about the causes behind this phenomenon, and the family will require additional support during this often emotional time. It is reasonable to believe, during a time of acute stress, that the mind will revert back to a period when the individual was best equipped to manage the excessive stress, felt the safest, happiest, or the strongest physically or emotionally. This survival mode provides a kind of disconnect from reality, and can help to distract and to relax the dying during their last few hours of life. There is no need to reorient the dying if this is a positive and comforting experience. Supporting their fantasy can often be the kinder and more compassionate option for care.

No matter what the cause for the delirium that occurs during the dying process, its presence can be upsetting to the family. It can be one of the first confirmations that a loved one is preparing to leave this world. All hope of meaningful communication can be lost and the emotional separation that results can be devastating for the family as they continue to crave one last lucid interaction. Family members will require additional education that the dying lack awareness of their behavior, that the stress of leaving them is likely just as intense, and that it is possible to be peacefully confused making the emotional separation from them more bearable.

GOALS OF CARE FOR THE DYING INDIVIDUAL WITH DELIRIUM

Close and Long (2012) suggested that the goals of care for the dying individual with delirium include:

- Maintaining safety, comfort, and well-being
- Identifying and treating reversible causes
- Educating the family on treatment and management
- Reassuring and holistically supporting both the patient and the family

Three types of delirium are identified in the literature: hypoactive, hyperactive, and mixed. Hypoactive delirium occurs in 86% of individuals diagnosed with terminal delirium. It is a sudden onset of unresponsiveness that can be easily confused with depression, oversedation, and emotional withdrawal (Ellershaw & Wilkinson, 2011; Ferrell & Coyle, 2010). The acute restlessness that can occur during the dying process is commonly called hyperactive delirium. Behavior that vacillates between acute restlessness and intermittent dispersions of somnolence is called mixed delirium. Hyperactive delirium is also commonly called terminal or agitated delirium and can vary from gentle moaning, and random continuous movement, to repetitive loud unreasonable requests, thrashing about, swearing, and futile attempts to get out of bed. The dying individual must be protected from injury and the family needs to be supported in their decision on how they want the delirium managed. Sedation will quiet the individual but could interfere with, or possibly eliminate, any chance of final meaningful communication.

The CARES tool suggests that the following treatment/strategies be considered.

- Give a trial dose of opioids to rule out pain. Often restlessness and delirium can be due to pain and the individual cannot verbalize the presence of this discomfort. A trial dose of an opioid can be given and the individual is then monitored for any improvement in mental status. This trial dose of opioids can be affective for all three forms of delirium.
- Assess for bladder distention and insert indwelling catheter if needed. Restlessness and delirium can be the result of painful bladder distention. Once this is resolved the individual will rest more comfortably and can often resume some meaningful interactions with their family.
- Assess for impaction if appropriate. When an individual is actively dying this option is usually omitted. For some individuals with chronic constipation, the family may request removal of the impaction so the dying individual can rest more comfortably. Rectal suppositories and subcutaneously injected methyl naltrexone can be given but should be weighed against time lost for final interactions with family.
- Consider use of antipsychotics such as haloperidol or chlorpromazine and/or benzodiazepines such as lorazepam or midazolam. The use of antipsychotics and benzodiazepines can reduce restlessness, repetitive activity, vocal outbursts, and allow the individual to rest more comfortably. It can also be effective in treating hypoactive delirium. Families should be informed that the medications may allow for some meaningful communication to occur, but in most instances the dying individual becomes more unresponsive. The use of sedation can be a difficult decision for some family members to make as there is also a risk that death could occur more quickly. The health care provider must supply

necessary education and assist the family in examining the risks versus the benefits of using antipsychotics and benzodiazepines. It is conceivable the dying individual, once sedated, can relax and allow death to occur naturally. The family must decide if allowing their loved one to suffer is worth potentially prolonging his or her dying with the hope there may be one, final, meaningful, verbal interaction. Families should be educated about the theory of intent, and asked to consider the needs of the dying individual over their own. The use of sedation is an individualized decision and does not guarantee a confused and combative individual will become coherent and that a meaningfully interact with their family. Families must be educated on the risks versus the benefits of sedation so an informed decision can be made.

- Maintain a calm environment. Minimizing stimulation from lights and loud noises can be calming and assist the dying individual to relax and become less restless. The nurse may suggest dimming the lights in the room, drawing the curtains, and reducing the flow of visitors. The family must ultimately decide what will be done and may again need gentle redirection to focus on the needs of the dying and not just their own agenda.

- Playing favorite music, talking softly stating "You are safe. We are with you. We love you"; maintaining the use of touch and presence, and the use of aromatherapy may help to calm and soothe the dying individual. These nonpharmaceutical methods can be extremely effective. The family should be reminded that hearing is believed to be the last sense lost in the dying process and familiar voices and sounds do appear to be a calming option for the treatment of delirium. Familiar and gentle soothing smells can also assist in calming a dying individual and should be considered.

Families of dying individuals with delirium may need to consider the possibility of unfinished business as a cause of restlessness and delirium. "Terminal anguish" is a phrase used to describe a dying individual's extreme emotional or spiritual suffering because of unresolved issues that do not respond to standard treatment. The health care provider should discuss with the family possible causes of this severe stress and anxiety and seek possible resolutions before resorting to deep sedation. Many issues can be resolved with the involvement of the family and the palliative care team. Weddings can be re-enacted, estranged family members can be flown in to resolve long-standing conflicts, and counseling and confessions can be heard by priests and end-of-life blessings can be provided by clergy.

Psychosocial concerns of dying individuals may also cause additional agitation and delirium-like symptoms and should be explored as part of an ongoing effort to calm and comfort the dying patient. The dying are often concerned about how their loved ones will manage without them and will struggle through their pain and suffering to remain alive for their benefit. The CARES tool suggests the nurse review with the family the importance of saying good-bye and giving their loved one permission to stop fighting. Family members may need to reassure the dying that they will be okay, and promise that specific family issues will be taken care of. This can be very difficult and the family members must be convincing so their dying loved one believes them and can let go and die peacefully. Health care providers must understand the importance of these activities and help family members in their efforts to comfort the dying. Providing reassurance for both the family and the dying individual is an extremely important contribution. It is easy to lose perspective and revert to self-protective behaviors. The health care provider may need to frequently redirect family members in an effort to maintain the desired focus of achieving the desired goals of the dying individual. Just the calm and empathetic presence of the nurse can be reassuring and help to effectively navigate the family through this very stressful time.

There are moments during delirium when the dying individual can become alert and oriented for hours or moments before he or she dies. There is no one plausible explanation for this occurrence and family members should be encouraged to enjoy the interaction for as long as it continues. Reassurances from health care providers are needed as this should be a time for the family to obtain further closure and additional memories of loving interactions that will sustain them through their grieving process.

An example of this dramatic change in consciousness occurred with a terminally ill individual named Paul. Paul was a 36-year-old gentleman dying of metastatic brain cancer, who was being cared for in an in-patient hospice facility. He was experiencing hyperactive delirium for the past week causing him to become restless and to shout random disconnected statements. His family sat at his bedside trying to soothe and calm him by reading aloud his favorite chapters from the *Hobbit*. His wife Mary was reading when suddenly Paul relaxed, opened his eyes, and from memory recited the same passage Mary had read. Mary stopped reading in disbelief and excitedly called for the nurse. Paul looked directly at Mary, smiled and said "Hi, Honey" and then yawned. The nurse entered the room and found Mary curled up next to Paul in his hospital bed with her head on his chest. Paul had his arm around Mary and was speaking softly to her.

The nurse introduced herself as Martha and asked how Paul was feeling as she performed a brief neurologic exam. Paul's left pupil was still blown, indicating significant brain damage, yet Paul was awake and laughing with his wife. Paul remained awake for another hour and then told his wife he was tired and needed a nap. Paul never woke up again, and died peacefully 3 days later.

The medical staff felt the swelling within Paul's brain must have diminished enough with dehydration that some brain function was restored, but hypothesized that the reduced pressure just provided more space for his brain tumor to shift and redistribute new pressure on Paul's brain stem to cause his death. Regardless of the cause, Paul and Mary were provided 3 precious hours together to state their love and to say good-bye.

When Paul fell back to sleep, Martha brought Mary a cup of tea and sat with her in silence. Mary was still very excited about the event and kept repeating how grateful she was for the time they had. Martha listened to her and nodded. Mary admitted she knew nothing had changed and that Paul was still dying, but she was grateful for the extra time. Martha agreed it was a beautiful gift, and it also helped the health care staff to see Paul awake and interacting. Martha also commented on how peaceful Paul was now.

A neurologic exam by the house physician found that both of Paul's pupils had blown and he was no longer arousable. Martha was grateful Paul was not at a large hospital where they would have taken him to imaging and x-ray to confirm just what transpired, and the precious time he had with his wife would have been lost. Mary sat holding her husband's hand and was aware he was finally at peace.

It is important for the health care provider to realize that if the dying individual is peaceful and calm, so will his or her family be. A nurse's expertise can cause an incident like Paul's to escalate out of control or else be taken as a gift that is supported and embraced. Education and the use of effective communication are essential to promote a peaceful dying experience. Families require assistance to transcend the sadness of losing a loved one to celebrating the individual and the time they had together. The health care provider plays an important role in educating and guiding the family through the dying process. Excellent listening skills and the use of a therapeutic presence are essential.

Research has shown the family needs the health care provider's presence and calm supportive demeanor to provide a normal point of reference as they continue to interact with the extensive stressors so prevalent with the dying process. Often these nontechnical skills are deemed insignificant and there is the implication that the need for nursing care is minimal when, in fact, the opposite is true. It is not easy for a nurse to be fully present and accept that he or she cannot fix, or take measures to correct, a medical situation. Often the greatest skill required for caring for the dying with delirium is to bear witness, maintain a therapeutic presence, and help the family focus on the individual and not the disease.

STEVEN'S SYMPTOM MANAGEMENT

The ongoing example of the care provided Steven as he died continues to emphasize concepts discussed in this chapter. Steven may have experienced hypoactive delirium during his dying process. He was unable to provide any verbal or nonverbal acknowledgment of his family and did not display any signs of physical suffering when first assessed. The parents were encouraged to remove their gloves and gowns and hold their son's hand and comfort him as they had done during his 20 years of life. Speaking softly to Steven was suggested and telling him of their love and the pride they felt having him as their son was encouraged. A short conversation evolved about Steven and his parents smiled for the first time as they talked about his childhood and how he hoped to become a nurse.

The tension in the room seemed to lessen as attention shifted to the stories being told. Steven's parents were able to take an emotional break from the stress they were enduring to celebrate their son. The tears continued, but now a sense of peace and acceptance was evolving. The nurses took turns sitting in silence as the mother held her son and gently rocked him against her.

Delirium and restlessness, no matter the cause, play an active role in disconnecting from the real world and advancing toward death. They provide a path toward closure, an opportunity to express feelings, and time to celebrate the dying as the special individual he once was. Delirium can be made peaceful with the use of appropriate medications and the reduction of irritating stimuli. Families need to be encouraged to be involved and help emphasize the dying individual that he is safe, loved, and supported.

There are so many wonders to the dying process. The gifts of memories and closure need to be encouraged. The dying with delirium and their families can still experience a loving and peaceful death. Skilled symptom management, the use of strong communication skills that focus on the celebration of the individual, and fully experiencing the time together can keep the presence of delirium from diminishing the opportunity for meaningful closure.

REFERENCES

Brajtman, S. (2005). Helping the family through the experience of terminal restlessness. *Journal of Hospice and Palliative Nursing, 7*(2), 73–81.

Close, J. F., & Long, C. O. (2012). Delirium: Opportunity for comfort in palliative care. *Journal of Hospice and Palliative Nursing, 14*(6), 386–394.

Ellershaw, J., & Wilkinson, S. (2011). *Care of the dying: A pathway to excellence* (2nd ed.). New York, NY: Oxford University Press.

Ferrell, B. R., & Coyle, N. (Eds.). (2010). *Oxford textbook of palliative nursing* (3rd ed.). New York, NY: Oxford University Press.

CHAPTER 10

Emotional and Spiritual Care

Spirituality is essential to the holistic health of patients, their families, and health care providers (Hutchinson, 2011). It addresses the "inner reality of human beings," and provides a deeper understanding of our life's purpose (p. 151). It cannot be easily defined, yet it is evident in the values and ethics of all individuals. Spirituality has an important role in patient care and impacts nursing theory, research, and education (Taylor, 2002). It is influenced by culture, religion, personal life philosophy, and can be equated with our very soul.

THE DIMENSIONS OF SPIRITUALITY

There are varying opinions on how spirituality should be defined and the impact religion and psychology can have on an individual's definition of spirituality. There are differing opinions on the extent religion plays, and on the acceptance that a person can be spiritual and not belong to an organized religion. Spirituality can be viewed as mystical and as a desire to be a part of something beyond the self. The variety of definitions can prompt lively debates with some responses more heated and passionate than others. Many of the discussions require an open mind and a nonjudgmental attitude. Often the role religion plays in an individual's personal sense of spirituality can obstruct maintaining an open and unbiased view of the spiritual needs of others. This is mirrored in the difficulties often found when caring for individuals with different beliefs, such as Wicca and devil worship. The extremes in worship practices can challenge some nurses as they will need to put aside their beliefs and provide care despite their religious differences.

The best methods to support an individual's spirituality require an understanding of the importance of being present, acting as a sounding board, and listening without judging. Spirituality is unique to every individual and reflects the very essence of who he or she is.

My philosophical understanding of spirituality can best be summarized by Puchalski and Ferrell's (2010) definition developed during a 2009 spirituality consensus conference: "Spirituality is the aspect of humanity that refers to the way individuals seek and express meaning and purpose, and the way they experience their connectedness to the moment, to self, to others, to nature and to the significant" (p.16).

I believe spirituality is a reflection of our soul. It is who we are at our deepest internal core. It is shaped by life experiences, religion, values, and the ethical standards that we have come to embrace as individuals. Our spirituality must be nurtured and respected as it affects our sense of dignity, self-worth, and purpose in life. It is who we are at our most vulnerable. Spirituality is not defined by our career, role in society, age, or ethnicity. Rather, spirituality is an expression of our purpose, value, dignity, and connectedness with others and to God.

Spirituality also reflects a multivariable human need that defies a single definition. Broadly defined, it is much more than just an individual's religious beliefs, in many cases religion may not play a part of defining one's spirituality, and for others it provides the very foundation for their personal values and identity (Puchalski & Ferrell, 2010). A common thread for most definitions of spirituality recognizes an individual's values, rituals, self-perceptions, and personal insights as unique aspects that define him or her and allows for "transcending the commonplace and searching their soul for deeper meaning" (Mauk & Schmidt, 2004, p. 3). Dossey, Keegan, Kolkmeier, and Guzzetta (1989) defined spirituality as:

> A broad concept that encompasses values, meaning, and purpose; one turns inward to the human traits of honesty, love, caring, wisdom, imagination, and compassion; existence of a quality of a higher authority, guiding spirit or transcendence that is mystical; a flowing, dynamic balance that allows and creates healing of body–mind–spirit, and may or may not involve organized religion. (p. 24)

Limitations of spirituality can be attributed to the difficulty that exists in defining its true meaning and importance. Spirituality remains confused with religiosity, psychology, and mysticism.

Spiritual patient care needs could be greatly compromised if holistic support remains based on religiosity. Often, the deeper meaning of spirituality is not explored beyond an individual's religious practices. Persons claiming no religious affiliation are at a greater disadvantage for holistic spiritual support because of the misunderstanding of the basic tenets of spirituality by health care providers.

RESEARCH AND SPIRITUALITY

Research validating the important role that spirituality plays in the lives of human beings is often discounted because of an inability to clearly differentiate study results from the effects of religion, psychology, and mysticism (Koenig, 2011).

Research continues to explore and attempt to clearly define spirituality. Koenig (2011) combined spirituality and religion as one entity in his research. He focused on exploring the human need for spiritual/religious beliefs and practices. Koenig's (2011) review of research studies on mental health noted 70% to 75% focused on the effects of religion, spirituality, and health. In 2010, there were 326 quantitative studies examining the relationship that exists between religion, spirituality, and well-being. The relationship between religion, spirituality, hope, and optimism was explored in 40 studies with 73% ($n = 29$) noting positive correlation between individuals with a strong religious and spiritual focus and the presence of hope and optimism in their lives. All studies comparing incidences of depression, self-esteem, personal control, suicidal ideation, and having a meaning and purpose in life found the more religious and spiritual an individual was the healthier he or she was physically, mentally, and socially (Koenig, 2011).

The strengths of the research can be found in the large number of studies, long periods of observation, different cultural groups studied, and the consistent results confirming the health benefits of religious and spiritual beliefs. Weaknesses in this research can be found in the 80% to 90% use of cross-sectional designs that cannot clearly define if the health state was attributable to the presence of religion and spirituality, or if the health state promoted religion and spirituality. Again, research did not strive to differentiate between religion and spirituality. Other weaknesses noted by Koenig (2011) include poor control of cofounders, small samples, use of faulty measures, and overinterpretation of findings.

Valuable research findings can be obtained on spirituality if they are clearly defined and conducted with integrity and objectivity. Research in the field of spirituality remains of great importance, as noted by Koenig (2011), but it must be separated from religion to be clearly understood:

> Given the role that religion and spirituality could play in preventing illness, speeding recovery, and motivating individuals to care for one another in the community (thereby reducing the need for expensive health services), research in this area will be of critical importance in addressing the escalating health-care costs in the United States and countries around the world. (p. x)

Embracing the importance of spirituality in the clinical setting will allow for the acceptance of the important role humanity plays in providing quality holistic patient focused care (Byock, 2012; Puchalski & Ferrell, 2010). It emphasizes the need for caregivers to treat their patients with dignity and respect, to recognize that they are more than a room number or a disease process, and are deserving of empathy and kindness. Often health care providers' greatest tool is their humanity (Cobb, Puchalski, & Rumbold, 2012). It can be more valuable than any technical skill or treatment, because the patient is made to feel valued and cared for (O'Brien, 1999; Puchalski & Ferrell, 2010). The positive atmosphere that results from incorporating support necessary to promote a patient's spirituality can greatly enhance the healing process and also comfort a patient as he or she journeys through the dying process (O'Brien, 2001).

Spirituality is often defined in nursing as what it is not (Pesut, 2013). It is not solely religion nor could it ever be any dehumanizing biomedical processes. It may very well be the defining factor that helps differentiate nursing from all other health care fields. Pesut (2013) suggests that supporting needs associated with spirituality evolved from nursing efforts to culturally relate to patients and families, provide some sense of morality in health care, and help patients and families find some sense of meaning associated with a disease process. Embracing a patient's spirituality transcends language and cultural barriers because the authentic human interaction required often melts away cultural and language differences, and helps health care providers find the "human connection even across seemingly chasms of differing beliefs" (Pesut, 2013, p. 6).

The protection and promotion of patients' self-esteem are essential to addressing their spirituality issues. Patients must be made to feel valued by treating them with dignity and respect, worthy because of a health care provider's willingness to take time to listen to them, honored because they are treated as unique individuals, and important because the health care provider desires to work with them to achieve their specific needs and goals of care (Byock, 2012; Puchalski & Ferrell, 2010; Taylor, 2002). Pesut (2013) noted that "spirituality was the unifying force that made us all the same despite differing beliefs" (p. 6).

REED'S THEORY OF SELF-TRANSCENDENCE AND SPIRITUALITY

Pamela Reed's middle-range Theory of Self-Transcendence can provide further insight into the importance of supporting an individual's spirituality and provides a focus for the CARES tool for care of the dying. Reed (1991a) defined self-transcendence as a "characteristic of developmental maturity requiring an expansion of self-boundaries and an orientation toward broadened life perspectives and purposes" (p. 64). She based her theory on deductive reformulation, life span developmental psychology, Rogers's conceptual system, clinical experience, and her empirical investigations.

Reed identified that individuals continue to develop throughout their life span and this process continues until death. She believed that as humans age they are less affected by time passing and more affected by the influences of their life experiences and events (Pesut, 2013; Reed, 2008). Reed theorized that the maintenance of mental health at end of life required the developmental phenomenon of self-transcendence. The Self-Transcendence theory addresses patients and their families' sense of compromised well-being at the end of life and the need to transcend those feelings and concerns to successfully support spirituality (Pesut, 2013). Self-transcendence provides the ability to find meaning from life's challenges and achieve a sense of well-being and wholeness (Reed, 2008).

The Theory of Self-Transcendence is based on two assumptions: human beings are multidimensional and capable of an expanded awareness of the world and themselves beyond their five senses, and human beings are cognitively drawn or possess a "developmental imperative" to seek a sense of well-being essential to self-transcendence (Reed, 2008). "Self-transcendence embodies experiences that connect rather than separate a person from self, others, and the environment" (p. 2178). It is an enhanced awareness and a broadening of life perspectives that is only obtainable through developmental maturity (Reed, 2008). Some expressions of self-transcendence noted by Reed include:

- Sharing wisdom with others
- Integrating of the physical changes of aging
- Accepting death as a part of life
- Finding spiritual meaning in life (Reed, 2008, p. 2206)

The Theory of Self-Transcendence has three major concepts. The first is the general assumptions about transcendence as previously discussed, the second is the theory of well-being, and the last major concept addresses vulnerability.

Well-being can be defined in numerous ways. It is often described as a feeling of wholeness and health, and is positively linked to the development of self-transcendence. Some indicators of well-being are equated with life satisfaction, positive self-esteem and self-concept, hopefulness, happiness, and life meaningfulness (Reed, 2008). Reed theorized that a state of well-being directly correlated with the ability to obtain self-transcendence.

Vulnerability was defined as an awareness of mortality, and the acceptance that difficult events will normally occur in a person's lifetime. When confronted with these issues, self-transcendence should naturally occur in the healthy individual. "Life events that heighten one's sense of mortality, inadequacy, or vulnerability can—if they do not crush the individual's inner self-trigger development, progress toward a renewed sense of identity and expanded self-boundaries" (Reed, 2008, p. 2215). A person's vulnerability is the catalyst to achieving self-transcendence. Common life events that evoke the sense of vulnerability include life crisis, chronic illness, aging, disability, parenting, childbirth, loss of a loved one, and career difficulties. When a life crisis occurs, self-transcendence can enhance a sense of well-being that allows for the transformation of the crisis into a healing and learning experience (Reed, 2008). This process has also been called post-traumatic growth. It is believed that it is when the heart is "broken," when an individual is most vulnerable, that they are the most open to spiritual growth and change (Wicks, 2006).

The transformation of a crisis to a healing and learning experience requires support of the individual's spirituality. Reed is a strong supporter of spirituality when caring for patients and their families. The concepts of transcendence, well-being, hopefulness, positive self-esteem, life satisfaction, and meaningfulness in life are all defining factors of an individual's spirituality.

Vulnerability is also a factor in determining the spirituality needs of patients and their families. A sense of vulnerability can be tempered, if not totally eliminated, if a patient's spiritual needs are met and self-transcendence is allowed to occur. The Theory of Self-Transcendence is based on the nurturing and support of a patient's spirituality.

PARSE'S THEORY OF HUMANBECOMING AND SPIRITUALITY

Another theory that supports self-transcendence is the Humanbecoming theory by Parse (1998). The ever-changing and unpredictable nature of human beings is explored and the need for nursing to bear witness to the individual health journey each patient experiences. Patients need their uniqueness acknowledged, to feel someone is really listening, and they need to feel they are emotionally supported (Maxwell Smith, 2010). When a nurse is attentively present it provides an opportunity for patients to contemplate and express how they define their health status, meanings in their life, and to feel they are being heard. Each patient has a unique perspective about his or her health. Parse theorized that health is cocreated within the universe of every human being, is specific to the individual, and cannot be quantified, or judged as good or bad. Parse defined health as "a personal commitment that each person lives incarnating his or her own value priorities" (Parse, 1998, p. 32).

Parse (1998) theorized humans mentally construct what is real for them based on multiple life experiences and interactions with different realms of the universe. She believes humans share their values through speaking, silence, moving, and being still. Her use of opposite poles of action reinforce the rhythmical patterns of the universe that are forever changing and evolving to influence human values and promote the growth of possibilities. "Humans change moment to moment as they actualize dreams and hopes through inventing new ways to propel beyond what is to what is not yet" (Parse, 1999, p. 8).

Parse's Theory of Humanbecoming is similar to Reeds's Theory of Self-Transcendence because both theories address:

- Emotional and cognitive growth that continues to occur until death
- Self-esteem that must be supported to enhance spirituality
- The need to feel valued and unique
- Individuals who must adjust and evolve with changes in their life and environment.

  - Parse theorized change influences human values and promotes a growth of possibilities
  - Reed theorized developmental maturity requires an expansion of self-boundaries and a broadening of life perspectives and purposes

- A desire to achieve a heightened state of existence.

  - Humanbecoming
  - Self-transcendence

The differences in the theories are more in the semantics and specific age group focus. Parse is more futuristic and addresses all levels of growth when exposed to change. Reed is more closely tied to spirituality, the elderly, the terminally ill, and the dying. She theorizes transcendence needs to occur to accept and rise above the hardships of dying and grief. Parse theorized humans must change and evolve to achieve what so far has not been attainable.

SELF-TRANSCENDENCE AND SPIRITUALITY

Pamela Reed's Theory of Self-Transcendence is based on spirituality. Self-transcendence requires the basic tenets of a well-supported spirituality. The individual must have a strong sense of self-worth, value, and purpose to transcend the grief and difficult life changes associated with the dying process.

Coward and Reed (1996) in "Self-Transcendence: A Resource for Healing at the End of Life" noted that supporting spirituality promotes expansion of self-boundaries to allow for healing. Healing was defined as finding meaning in an adverse situation, promoting a renewed sense of self, and the expansion of a sense of wholeness. The perspectives are considered very important in the terminally ill as they can assist with subjective well-being. This well-being allows the individual to look beyond themselves and gain insight into meanings and purpose regarding life and death. Health care providers must assist their dying patients with establishing a connectiveness with the transpersonal to achieve an increased awareness and integration of all dimensions of being.

Reed's (1986) article, "Religiousness Among Terminally Ill and Healthy Adults," reviewed research obtained from 57 terminally ill and 57 healthy adults on the role religion played in their sense of well-being. Religiousness, much like spirituality, was defined as "the perception of one's beliefs and behaviors that express a sense of relatedness to spiritual dimensions or to something greater than the self" (p. 36). Well-being was defined as "a sense of satisfaction with one's current life" (p. 36). The study concluded that being both terminally ill and female provided the greatest incidence of religiousness, and older terminally ill patients had a significantly higher sense of well-being than younger patients. Awareness of a limited life span may be the greatest contributor to religiousness.

Reed (1987) noted in a study of 300 adults titled "Spirituality and Well-Being in Terminally Ill Hospitalized Adults" that spirituality was a substantial human experience that did not differ significantly between hospitalized terminally ill and nonterminally ill patients. Spirituality was associated with a reduced fear of death, reduced discomfort, improved emotional adjustment, and decreased loneliness. Spirituality was defined as the culmination of personal views and behaviors that evolved according to life experiences and events allowing for a connectiveness to something greater than the self. Spirituality was identified as an essential component for the ability to achieve the mental task of transcendence defined as "a level of awareness that exceeds ordinary physical boundaries and limitations" (p. 335). The biological and physical changes associated with dying caused individuals to utilize spirituality as a primary method of coping to achieve a sense of well-being. A small but consistent relationship was confirmed between spirituality and a sense of well-being for the terminally ill in this study.

Reed's (1991a) article "Self-Transcendence and Mental Health in Oldest-Old Adults" explored the impact of self-transcendence on well-being for older adults. Fifty-five older adults, ages 80 to 97, residing at independent living facilities participated in the mixed-methods study. The theoretical framework was based on life span development. It addressed the human need for connectiveness with self and the environment. Four patterns of self-transcendence were identified as important for a sense of well-being: generativity, an altruistic motivated desire to help others and family; introjectivity, a desire to focus on inner-directed activities and available environmental resources such as hobbies, lifelong learning, and spiritual reflection; temporal integration, the mental review of past, present, and the anticipation of future plans and accomplishments; and body-transcendence, the acceptance and integration of body and cognitive changes into current lifestyle. Results of the study supported previous research that found a direct relationship between self-transcendence and mental health.

Reed (1991b) noted, in the article "Toward a Nursing Theory of Self-Transcendence: Deductive Reformation Using Developmental Theories," the need to develop theories addressing developmental phenomenon and the promotion of a sense of well-being in later life. Nursing and psychology theories of development were merged to develop a nursing theory about self-transcendence. Self-transcendence was identified as a characteristic of developmental maturity identified by an expansion of self-boundaries, broadening life perspectives, and an enhanced sense of purpose and self-worth. The identification of the process of self-transcendence provides proof that human beings continue to cognitively evolve until death. The theory proposes that self-transcendence occurs most often with an increased awareness of mortality usually found when confronting a terminal illness. The ability to transcend the challenges of a terminal illness directly correlates with well-being. This theory directly impacts the important role nurses play in the care and support of a patient's spirituality, especially when caring for the terminally ill.

Reed (1992) in "An Emerging Paradigm for the Investigation of Spirituality in Nursing" noted that spirituality has long been a focus of nursing practice. Nursing regards spirituality as a human phenomenon essential to health and well-being. Spirituality addresses the ability to derive meaning through three dimensions of relatedness and connectivity: the interpersonal, a connection to self; the intrapersonal, a connection to others and the environment; and the transpersonal, a connection to the unseen, God, or a higher power. This spiritual connectiveness allows for the transcendence of self that results in an increased sense of self-worth, personal empowerment, and "endows the ordinary with extraordinary meaning" (p. 350). Spirituality is a broad concept that is difficult to measure. It is a multidimensional concept with a vertical dimension of connectiveness and a horizontal dimension of relatedness to the environment both socially and physically. It crosses traditional science boundaries and requires a "strong dose of humility" to study (p. 355).

All articles reviewed provided a direct relationship with an individual's spirituality and his or her ability to attain self-transcendence. The awareness of mortality was found to be a significant trigger to cause an individual to draw upon his or her spiritual strengths. These spiritual strengths provided the emotional and cognitive resources necessary to transcend the fears and obstacles most commonly found with the terminally ill and dying. Self-transcendence was found to be a common end-of-life goal and an essential component to achieve a sense of well-being.

The need to transcend the overwhelming issues inherent during the dying process for both the patient and his or her family requires extensive spiritual support. The CARES tool specifically addresses the emotional and spiritual needs of a dying patient and his or her family. The tool was developed with a focus on holistic support that nurtures and promotes self-transcendence. Spirituality needs that must be addressed to allow for self-transcendence include feelings of being valued, worthy of help, respected, listened to, and comforted. A sense of well-being can flourish when spiritual needs are supported and self-boundaries are expanded.

The state of self-transcendence as described by Reed (2008) involves the interpersonal growth of:

- Self-boundaries, which would allow for a greater awareness of one's philosophy, values, and dreams
- The ability to relate to others and one's environment
- Temporal capacity, to allow for the integration of one's past and future in a way that has meaning for the present
- Transpersonal capacity, to allow for a connection with dimensions beyond the typically discernable world

The CARES tool is based on the need to support a patient and his or her family's spirituality. All five sections of the tool address the most common symptom management needs of the dying and those of individuals providing their care. Each symptom has a foundation in spirituality and was selected to assist in the transcendence beyond physical and psychological requirements to achieve the much broader sense of peace and well-being.

EMOTIONAL AND SPIRITUAL SUPPORT

The "E" in the CARES tool incorporates concepts of emotional and spiritual support. It directly relates to the theoretical foundation of the CARES tool: to promote and support the achievement of self-transcendence. The section emphasizes the importance of humanity and encourages communication, active listening, and supportive presence.

Actual prompts and suggestions provided in the CARES tool to assist in meeting the emotional and spiritual needs of the dying include:

- Focus on caring for the soul
- Provide emotional, psychosocial, and cultural support
- The need to know available resources and how to access them
- Recognize that health care staff may be in need of emotional and spiritual support, too
- Always work to retain the patient's dignity and feelings of value
- Be aware of the different methods of grieving
- The importance of good communication skills, and ensure all parties involved are "on the same page"

- Always refer back to the family, they should remain the driving force for care
- Never assume you know what the family wants, always confirm with them directly
- Provide as much information as the family requests
- Continue to clarify and follow established goals of care
- Maintain the family's privacy needs
- Continue to provide a supportive presence, and just be with the family
- Suggest the family provide their loved one's favorite music, clothing, foods, and so on—anything they feel could be comforting
- Consider bringing in a favorite pet or providing a favorite activity even if it is amended to the confines of the hospital room
- Support family rituals by obtaining any needed equipment or available personnel
- Remember your humanity is needed most of all. Be present, compassionate, and nonjudgmental
- Monitor the family and encourage breaks, make food and drink readily available
- Remember, you cannot take away their pain; acknowledge their emotion and be present

STEVEN'S SYMPTOM MANAGEMENT

Steven continued to become less responsive and was in the final hours to moments of his young life. Emotional and spiritual support continued for the parents as described in Chapter 9 on restlessness and delirium. It is important to note that much of the content found in the individual sections of comfort, airway, restlessness and delirium, emotional and spiritual care, and self-care overlap and do not exclusively belong in only one section of the tool. Spirituality is a classic example as all sections of the CARES tool have a foundation in spirituality. If symptoms are not controlled, the dying and their families cannot successfully transcend the sadness and grief associated with dying and progress to celebrating the life lived and the gift of having known this individual.

Steven's parents obtained emotional support by being allowed to actively participate in the care of their son. The ability to decide what comfort measures were needed, whether to increase the morphine, or when to provide oral suctioning gave them a small sense of control in an uncontrollable time.

Staff addressed Steven respectfully by name, and the parents were aware of how emotional many of the nurses had become as Steven's life was ending. They verbalized their gratefulness over the loving care their son received and appreciated how kind everyone was to them. The primary nurse sat with the family and listened to more stories about Steven and continued to reassure the parents that Steven was not suffering.

The goal in providing emotional and spiritual support is to help the dying and their families celebrate life, the time they had together, and their ability to transcend the confines of dying to embrace a sense of peace, support, well-being, and acceptance. This is ultimately the overall goal of the CARES tool.

REFERENCES

Byock, I. (2012). *The best care possible: A physician's quest to transform care through end of life*. New York, NY: Avery.

Cobb, M., Puchalski, C. M., & Rumbold, B. (Eds.). (2012). *Oxford textbook of spirituality in healthcare*. New York, NY: Oxford University Press.

Coward, D. D., & Reed, P. G. (1996). Self-transcendence: A resource for healing at the end of life. *Issues in Mental Health Nursing, 17*, 275–288.

Dossey, B. M., Keegan, L., Kolkmeier, G., & Guzzetta, C. E. (Eds.). (1989). *Holistic health promotion: A guide for practice*. Rockville, MD: Aspen.

Hutchinson, T. A. (2011). *Whole person care: A new paradigm for the 21st century*. New York, NY: Springer Publishing.

Koenig, H. G. (2011). *Spitituality & health research: Methods, measurement, statistics, and resources*. West Conshohocken, PA: Templeton Press.

Mauk, K. L., & Schmidt, N. A. (2004). *Spiritual care in nursing practice*. Philadelphia, PA: Lippincott, Williams & Wilkins.

Maxwell Smith, S. (2010). Humanbecoming: Not just a theory—It is a way of being. *Nursing Science Quarterly, 23*(3), 216–219.

O'Brien, M. E. (1999). *Spirituality in nursing: Standing on holy ground*. Sudbury, MA: Jones and Bartlett.

O'Brien, M. E. (2001). *The nurse's calling: A Christian spirituality of caring for the sick*. Mahwah, NJ: Paulist Press.

Parse, R. R. (1998). *The human becoming school of thought*. Thousand Oaks, CA: Sage Publications.

Parse, R. R. (1999). *NLN press illuminations: The human becoming theory in practice and research*. Boston, MA: Jones and Bartlett.

Pesut, B. (2013). Nursings' need for the idea of spirituality. *Nursing Inquiry, 20*(1), 5–10.

Puchalski, C. M., & Ferrell, B. R. (2010). *Making health care whole: Integrating spirituality into patient care*. West Conshohocken, PA: Templeton Press.

Reed, P. G. (1986). Religiousness among terminally ill and healthy adults. *Research in Nursing & Health, 9*, 35–41.

Reed, P. G. (1987). Spirituality and well-being in terminally ill hospitalized adults. *Research in Nursing & Health, 10*, 335–344.

Reed, P. G. (1991a). Self-transcendence and mental health in oldest-old adults. *Nursing Research, 40*(1), 5–11.

Reed, P. G. (1991b). Toward a nursing theory of self-transcendence: Deductive reformulation using developmental theories. *Advanced Nursing Science, 13*(4), 64–77.

Reed, P. G. (1992). An emerging paradigm for the investigation of spirituality in nursing. *Research in Nursing & Health, 15,* 349–357.

Reed, P. G. (2008). Theory of self-transcendence. In M. J. Smith & P. R. Liehr (Eds.), *Middle range theory for nursing* (2nd ed., chapter 6) [Kindle edition]. New York, NY: Springer Publishing.

Taylor, E. J. (2002). *Spiritual care: Nursing theory, research, and practice.* Upper Saddle River, NJ: Prentice Hall.

Wicks, R. J. (2006). *Overcoming secondary stress in medical and nursing practice: A guide to professional resilience and personal well-being.* New York, NY: Oxford University Press.

CHAPTER 11

Self-Care

The final topic of the CARES tool addresses the importance of self-care for the health care provider. Caring for the dying and their families can be very stressful—physically, emotionally, and spiritually. Issues of moral distress, burnout, and compassion fatigue are common. The sharing and gaining of insight into personal frustrations, sadness, and loss can assist the caregiver to find meaning and personal growth from his or her experiences. Often, just the act of converting feelings into words can be healing.

THE WORK OF ROBERT WICKS AND SELF-CARE

The work of Robert Wicks (2006) is the reference utilized for much of the recommended self-care techniques discussed in this chapter. Wicks is a psychologist and a professor at Loyola College in Maryland. He has published over 40 books to assist professionals dealing with clients experiencing tragedy and loss. His work was discovered by this author while attending an Association of Death Educators and Councilors (ADEC) National Conference in 2014. ADEC's membership is primarily composed of social workers, psychologists, and spiritual councilors. The lectures from the conference provided great insight into methods of self-care used by these professionals and with first responders, firemen, policemen, and grief counselors.

Nursing programs are just beginning to acknowledge the role professional grieving plays in the lives of many nurses, so it is only logical to draw on established techniques used by other professionals exposed to various forms of tragedy and sadness on a daily basis. Nursing students are cautioned against overt displays of emotion. When in school, becoming tearful and/or crying was discouraged and was considered unprofessional or the result of a loss of self-control. Nurses were reminded to be professional and to not allow emotions to affect their care and judgment. This work ethic has greatly contributed to the loss of personal resilience, the development of secondary stress and burnout, and the exodus of many compassionate individuals from the nursing profession. The fact that nurses are human beings with human emotions was ignored. Nurses were made to feel weak or inadequate if they displayed any emotional response to the death of an individual under their care.

Nurses were held to the same standards as many health care professionals, and crying or overt demonstrations of grief were believed to only amplify failure. Other nurse coworkers did not provide comfort or support as they were unprepared how to assist in a grieving process that was not deemed acceptable, or was too painful for them to acknowledge. Nurses learned to grieve in the silence of a near-by restroom and would "pull themselves together" out of sheer personal willpower until one day their willpower was depleted. No techniques to restore or promote personal resilience were provided. Nurses risked disapproval from their peers if they openly sought support, and they would eventually become distant or avoid close interactions with individuals under their care, opt to transfer to another areas with less personal contact, or resign (Wicks, 2006).

Wicks (2012) shares that effective self-care requires a daily commitment. The transition to provide healthy self-care practices in the work setting continues to be slow and could never be specific enough to address the needs of all individuals. As a professional group, there still remains a stigma to professional grieving and as always, change will be slow. Wicks used the analogy of it being easier to "protect your feet by putting on slippers rather than to carpet the world," in the keynote address he gave at the 2014 ADEC conference in Baltimore, Maryland. He encouraged health care providers to seek their own methods of emotional and psychological support and make them part of a daily practice as he noted the development of burnout was a "slow insidious process and not the result of just one event" (Wicks, 2014).

Wicks believed there must be a focus on mindfulness. There must be a willingness by health care providers to consciously explore the day's events and their personal impact on the individual. It is important to view the events only in the present. The caregiver must stay in the here-and-now to successfully separate a distressing event from a past personal experience. Wicks (2014) described these techniques as living "only a short distance from the body."

The need to remain in the present is emphasized as health care providers must attempt to discover what personal factors contributed to their emotional responses. An example of this process is as follows: A health care provider takes time out to get a cup of coffee and explore her grief response after being informed that a person under her care had just died at another facility.

The news was emotionally painful for the nurse and she was quickly brought to tears. She shared her sadness with some coworkers but none of them remembered the man. The nurse began to feel both embarrassed at her perceived loss of control and angry. She felt alone, ashamed at how emotional she became, and abandoned because no one seemed to share or acknowledge her loss. She wanted to shout that a beautiful man was now dead and she couldn't do anything to prevent it, but no one else seemed to care. So, she got a cup of coffee and took some time to sit outside and process her feelings.

Daily emotional inventories taught this nurse to recall some important lessons learned from previous self-care lectures. The nurse was aware that health care providers must:

1. Be realistic. They cannot allow themselves to believe they are placed on a pedestal by the individuals under their care. They are not all-knowing or all-powerful.

2. Acknowledge that a power greater than their abilities or intentions will ultimately determine the fate of the individual.

3. Find comfort in knowing they did their very best.

4. Learn to celebrate the journey and the opportunity they were given when special individuals come into their lives.

5. Identify what parallels or issues of a death are being drawn to cause overidentification.

6. Stay in the present and remain only a short distance from their body. Take the time to separate their own personal issues from what actually happens.

7. Identify, explore, and work through personal issues that surface with the death of an individual under their care. This process can be painful but, ultimately, if done successfully and with professional help if necessary, it will result in personal growth. It is when the heart is most broken that we are in the best position to let new knowledge in, and forever change our perspectives on life and who we are as human beings (Wicks, 2006).

8. Identify some meaning, some growth obtained from the experience, and remember:

   . . . when all of life—both the perceived good and bad is faced directly with a sense of openness, life's promises are more fully realized. Moreover, this is not only important for the person experiencing the struggles but also for those they may touch after absorbing the new lessons learned about gratitude, impermanence/the frailty of life, simplicity, meaning-making, and compassion (Wicks, 2012, p. i).

The nurse focused on staying in the present. She became aware of the parallels she unconsciously drew between the individual who had died and her brother who was near the same age and was now recovering from a stroke. The nurse realized she was having some anticipatory grief regarding her brother and overidentifying with the family as they grieved for this very lovely man, who was so much like her brother, and who she was lucky enough to get to know.

She began to explore how realistic her expectations of herself were when no chemotherapy or radiation could halt the progression of his cancer. The nurse knew she did everything in her power to make him comfortable, to advocate for his needs, and to support his family. A sense of inner peace began to evolve with the acceptance that she had done her best.

Through a few more tears the nurse began to celebrate the opportunity she was given to care for this man and to get to know him and his family. She remembered her last interaction with him as he sat in a wheelchair and began to cry while resting his head against her. The nurse took pride in his comfort to be so vulnerable with her and for the opportunity she was given to say good-bye. The nurse knew in her heart she was a better person for having known him and was grateful for this beautiful gift.

Self-care is not easy. Health care professionals must view it as a daily priority and not hesitate because the process can be emotionally painful. This pain should not be avoided because it will accumulate until burnout becomes unavoidable. Accepting the presence of our emotional pain and committing to work to understand it is one of the best methods to achieve self-awareness. This process is what Wicks (2012) called "riding the dragon":

> By "facing the dragons of reality and truth" about our lives, much unforeseen growth, depth and promise becomes possible. It is not easy to face our lives at times. No one wants to experience, and it is not easy to face, loss, trauma, serious stress, and loneliness. This is very true. However, if we can learn to ride our dragons rather than run, hide from, or attack them, it can be transforming. (pp. ii–iii)

Self-awareness is essential for self-care. It provides a necessary level of comfort for health care providers to be human and to expect some personal emotional response to the death of individuals and for the grieving families under their care. It allows the nurse to separate his or her personal issues about death and dying from what is actually occurring. This allows the nurse to be compassionate and involved in care and helps him or her not to overidentify or choose to avoid becoming involved out of fear of losing emotional control.

Wicks's recommendation for a daily review of events is an important component to maintaining professional resiliency. The CARES tool also suggests nurses utilize palliative/supportive services if available and to participate in group reviews and debriefings, as discussed in detail in Chapter 21. Group support can assist with professional grieving and promote emotional health by:

- Formally acknowledging the stressful event and thanking supportive team members
- Reviewing what went well and what challenges need to be addressed from the varying perspectives of the participants
- Sharing bereaved family comments
- Addressing moral distress issues and finding they are not unique to just one individual
- Expressing issues of death anxiety and obtaining support and comfort from your peers
- Exploring challenges and privileges of assisting a fellow human being through the dying process
- Acknowledging the spiritual impact of witnessing a death
- Exploring how an individual's care made a difference
- Reviewing effective communication techniques, available resources, and support

Self-care must include mindfulness or self-awareness of the personal baggage we all carry. Daily reviews are essential for addressing the many stressors that can accumulate to slowly cause the health care professional to succumb to secondary stress, grief, hopelessness, and burnout. Group support from peers, staying in the present, and accepting the limitations of the care a nurse can provide can all assist in maintaining personal resiliency. When we stop running from the emotional pain caring for the dying can cause, and choose to "ride the dragon," it can open the health care provider to many unique lessons about his or her own personal strengths and how helplessness and loss can be faced with dignity, how being vulnerable can open an individual to self-acceptance, and how humility can be the very door that leads to compassion (Wicks, 2012).

The work of Wicks is strongly recommended to help health care providers learn how to effectively obtain self-care.

REFERENCES

Wicks, R. J. (2006). *Overcoming secondary stress in medical and nursing practice: A guide to professional resilience and personal well-being.* New York, NY: Oxford University Press.

Wicks, R. J. (2012). *Riding the dragon: Ten lessons for inner strength in challenging times.* Notre Dame, IN: Sorin Books.

Wicks, R. J. (2014). *Key note address: Riding the dragon.* Paper presented at the ADEC 2014 National Conference, Baltimore, MD.

See the Association for Death Education and Counseling (ADEC) website: www.ADEC.org

PART III

Foundation and Use

CHAPTER 12

Theories of Self-Transcendence and Structure of Caring

The use of nursing theories helps to better define the focus of the CARES tool and to establish the intent for the tool's usage. Two nursing theories helped to guide the development of the CARES tool and provided the desired focus on communication and hope that the CARES tool was designed to emphasize. Pamela Reed's middle-range Theory of Self-Transcendence and Kristen M. Swanson's Structure of Caring provided a guiding light to clearly define the very soul of the CARES tool.

SELF-TRANSCENDENCE

Reed (1991) focused on aging and the elderly when she defined self-transcendence as a "characteristic of developmental maturity requiring an expansion of self-boundaries and an orientation toward broadened life perspectives and purposes" (p. 64). Her definition of self-transcendence could apply to any expansion of the self that incorporates new perspectives, results in holistic growth, and promotes spiritual advancement of the individual.

Reed extended her theoretical emphasis when she concluded that the process of adapting to the many challenges inherent to a terminal disease requires the same basic tenets of self-transcendence as identified for the elderly (Pesut, 2013; Reed, 2008). Terminally ill individuals, such as the frail elderly, must have a sense of their own value and self-worth to transcend the often humiliating dependence on others for basic care and the resulting perceived loss of identity. This can be lessened by their families and health care providers through legacy work, review of life events, recognition of contributions to others, and through basic acts of respect and kindness.

The developmental phenomenon of self-transcendence is essential for the maintenance of mental health at the end of life. The dying must identify that they are so much more than their disease.

The self-transcendence theory addresses the concerns the dying individual and his or her family have over issues such as changing life roles and duties, and preparation for a life without each other. This compromised sense of well-being must transcend feelings of loss and despair and successfully support the spiritual needs of the dying individual and his or her family (Pesut, 2013). Self-transcendence provides the ability to find meaning from life's challenges and achieve a sense of well-being and wholeness (Reed, 2008).

Nurses play a crucial role in promoting self-transcendence as they are in the best position to nurture and promote individuals' use of their inner resources such as faith in a higher being, acceptance of their life course, and identification of their own inner strength and resources. The terminally ill may have physical and emotional symptoms such as pain, depression, and anxiety. The dying should be well palliated to fuel their inner strength and promote the development of self-transcendence.

With skillful symptom management, dying individuals can focus on issues such as how they want to be remembered, what they have accomplished, and how their life has made a difference. This form of legacy work will often assist in the search for meaning and re-inforce an individual's sense of self-value and worth. Self-transcendence can be a challenge to achieve as many individuals can become negative and self-punishing because of feelings that they have not accomplished anything of value in their life. The nurse, again, is in an opportune position to intervene as he or she can reframe events shared by a dying patient and identify specific aspects of pride to promote the human need for positive self-esteem, feelings of value and worth, and a belief that his or her life contributed in some small way to further mankind.

Simple acts such as knocking before entering a room, calling the individual by his or her name, actively listening, and encouraging clear defining of goals of care all imply an acknowledgment of the dying individual's uniqueness and value. It is through these basic actions caregivers' demonstrate their humanity, empathy, and compassion.

The Theory of Self-Transcendence was discussed in depth in Chapter 10. To review, Reed (2008) based her theory on two assumptions: (a) human beings are multidimensional and capable of an expanded awareness of the world and themselves beyond their five senses and (b) human beings are cognitively drawn or possess a "developmental imperative" to seek a sense of well-being essential to self-transcendence.

There must be an enhanced sense of self-awareness that occurs to allow the dying and their families to submit to the inevitable and accept their vulnerability. The nurse plays an essential role in nurturing this vulnerable grieving state to allow for the spiritual growth that can occur if meaning can be associated with the suffering they are enduring. Evidence-based symptom management must be provided for individuals to focus their energies on achieving this meaning and to strive for self-transcendence.

The dying and their families must be given a sense that they are valued and respected by the nurse and primary caregivers to find the inner strength necessary to complete their final journey. If the assistance is compassionate and respectful, the vulnerable individual and his or her family can achieve a sense of well-being and transcend the fears of the dying process and personal suffering.

STRUCTURE OF CARING

The second middle-range nursing theory to influence the development of the CARES tool is the Structure of Caring, developed by Swanson in 1991. There are five common caring processes or features to this theory that identify components of a caring relationship. The five components are maintaining belief, knowing, being with, doing for, and enabling (Swanson, 1993).

Swanson (1993) defines caring as "a nurturing way of relating to a valued other toward whom one feels a personal sense of commitment and responsibility" (p. 354). This definition of caring can be readily applied to the professional relationship that exists between the nurse and the dying individual he or she is caring for. The "personal sense of commitment and responsibility" portion of the caring definition could be directly applied to the important nursing role of acting as an advocate for the needs of the individuals under his or her care.

The first of the five components of the Structure of Caring theory addresses maintaining belief. Swanson notes maintaining belief is the foundation of nurse caring, and is demonstrated by the belief in the ability of individuals to transcend negative events and find meaning and a future focus with their assistance. This belief is also one of the basic tenets of Reed's Theory of Self-Transcendence. There must be a desire or human need to overcome adversity and the nurse can play a pivotal role in the achievement of this goal. The goal of the dying most commonly is to achieve a peaceful death.

Another component of the Structure of Caring theory is knowing. Swanson defines knowing as the desire to fully understand events and issues from the perspective of the individual under the care of the nurse. There is an avoidance of assumptions or beliefs, and the individual's identified needs and concerns will be utilized to drive his or her care. Knowing can only be achieved through open and honest communication. The dying need to have their concerns heard and be clearly understood so holistic support and treatment can be provided. An individual's concerns are unique and are heavily influenced by his or her culture, life experiences, and spirituality. Nurses are cautioned to know themselves so their own beliefs and biases do not limit their care. True knowing is necessary to promote well-being.

The next component of the Structure of Caring theory is being with. This component references the need for the nurse to be physically and emotionally present. Therapeutic presence allows for individuals under the nurse's care to fully express themselves. Meanings, life experiences, fears, and concerns can be readily expressed, and the nurse can convey acceptance, and diminish any fears of abandonment. Swanson (1993) notes the time given to provide this authentic presence also conveys that the individual is truly being listened to. "In many ways to be with another is to give simply of the self and to do so in such a way the one cared for realizes the commitment" (p. 355).

Nurses are cautioned that the need for self-care should be observed, because the opportunity to be open and obtain admission to the close inner circle of emotional and spiritual support required by the dying and their families can have an emotional toll on the nurse. The need for nurses to develop methods of self-care are encouraged because the closeness required for the component of "being with" can result in overidentification and secondary stress syndrome. Nurses are encouraged to learn to effectively support each other.

Another component of the Structure of Caring theory is "doing for." It shares the very definition of nursing. Swanson (1993) quoted Virginia Henderson's definition of nursing as:

> The unique function of the nurse is to assist the individual, sick or well, in the performance of those activities contributing to health or its recovery (or to a peaceful death) that he would perform unaided if he had the necessary strength, will, or knowledge. And to do this in such a way as to help him gain independence as rapidly as possible. (p. 356)

"Doing for," is simply the nurse doing for others what they cannot do for themselves. It is a purposeful action to preserve an individual's wholeness. Swanson (1993) cautions the nurse not to confuse actions based on their convenience, in the same way as those actions that address the specific needs of a patient, as "doing for" behaviors. Doing-for behaviors preserve an individual's dignity, comfort, and protect him or her from harm. They can also be helping behaviors as when a nurse arranges a support group or provides information and guidance about resources and programs to assist in achieving expressed needs. In the case of a dying patient, if a daughter expresses regret over no longer having tea with her mother, and the nurse arranges tea to be brought into the room, this behavior can be deemed "doing for."

Enabling is the final component of the Structure of Caring theory. It addresses the need for nurses to facilitate "others passage through life transitions and unfamiliar events" (Swanson, 1993, p. 356). Enabling includes teaching and coaching, supporting and encouraging the achievement of specific goals, providing alternatives to consider and feedback, and validating another's feelings and purpose to promote a sense of well-being. Caution must be exercised by the caregiver to ensure that his or her behavior is in the best interest of the individual he or she is helping. It is essential that efforts are applied to attain their goals and wishes and not those of the caregiver or nurse. Nurses' intent should be to nurture and promote transcendence; their behavior should be selfless and directed to assist in the achievement of the individual's goals.

STEVEN'S PEACEFUL DEATH

As expressed throughout this chapter, the nurse plays a crucial role in the achievement of self-transcendence for the dying and their families. In the case of Steven, the case we continue to address throughout this book, we found many opportunities to help Steven and his family transcend the emotional and physical suffering they were experiencing.

Steven was in nursing school and knew that his lung function was worsening. He communicated openly and honestly with his oncologist. She established a good rapport with Steven and his family. They were aware of the limited treatment options and Steven chose to travel and be with his friends and family until he could no longer care for himself. He established his goals of care to include a death without physical suffering. He confided that the fear of suffocation disturbed him the most. His oncologist assured Steven and his family that she would not let him suffer. She shared her plan to place Steven on supportive oxygen therapy and agreed with Steven not to intubate and place him on a ventilator. Steven made it clear he did not want to prolong his dying and he wanted to live out the time he had without the use of life support equipment.

The frank discussions about his death greatly disturbed Steven's mother. She agonized over the fact that nothing could be done to stop the inevitable death of her son. She respected Steven's wishes and worked to put his needs above her own. The oncologist's openness and skillful communication provided the necessary exchange of information, hopes, and desires for Steven and his family to be clearly understood.

Steven and his family's path to self-transcendence could be explained as follows.

- Steven's immediate fears of suffocation were diminished by his oncologist's reassurances thus allowing him to focus on establishing his goals of care.
- Steven was given emotional support by family and friends that allowed him to harness his inner strength to focus on visiting friends and saying good-bye.

- Steven was always listened to, treated with respect: his desire for privacy and to retain his dignity was always closely adhered to. He wanted to wear his ball cap 24 hours a day, have ice cream any time he wanted, and to never have information about his condition withheld. All of his requests were honored. Because of this, Steven focused his energies on spending time with his family and friends. He made legacy pillows, wrote letters, and made recordings for his family to watch after he died.

- Steven felt valued and loved by the nursing staff as evidenced by the close relationships he formed, the staff's willingness to spend time with Steven even on their days off, and the staff's desire to plan a Christmas party with Steven.

Steven declined rapidly and was unable to attend the Christmas party he helped plan. Throughout his illness and now during his final journey, Steven was treated as a unique individual and never as a room number or diagnosis. Nurses advocated for him to receive effective symptom management that included the addition of lorazepam and morphine delivered by an IV pump, as he became more anxious about his shortness of breath. He was reassured, and between the nursing staff and his family, he was never left alone.

Steven became progressively unresponsive over the next 24 hours. Staff continued to address him by name and to explain all procedures before attempting. They sought the parent's wishes regarding care and never assumed they wanted to be interrupted for turning, baths, or treatments. The parents were closely monitored by the staff to ensure they were getting their meals and rest. This atmosphere of compassion and support allowed the family to focus on their dying son and not expend essential energy worrying about personal needs. Steven's parents were supported by their clergy and the staff. There were tears, emotional support, and hand holding was freely provided. Steven and his parents were at their most vulnerable and, according to Reed, were the most open to self-transcendence. All was done to keep Steven comfortable, and to help his family feel supported, honored, and valued as they journeyed through the final death vigil.

Swanson and Reed both acknowledge the important role the nurse plays in the nurturing and maintenance of self-esteem. The dying and their families must feel valued, respected, and protected to allow for hope and self-esteem to flourish. Only then can individuals overcome adversity and transcend their fears because of the maintenance of belief behaviors. The nurse demonstrates knowing behaviors when he or she strives to identify the specific needs of the individuals in his or her care, and works to provide the resources necessary to accomplish his or her specific goals. The very act of trying to provide for these identified needs further promotes self-esteem for the dying patient and his or her family.

The therapeutic presence of the nurse helps to diminish fears associated with vulnerability and abandonment. The nurse's very focus should be to champion the unique needs of the dying and their families. Such supportive behaviors enable the dying and their families to therapeutically grieve and achieve the support they need to experience a peaceful death. Again, this is accomplished by promoting and supporting the individual's sense of self-worth.

REFERENCES

Pesut, B. (2013). Nursing's need for the idea of spirituality. *Nursing Inquiry, 20*(1), 5–10.

Reed, P. G. (1991). Toward a nursing theory of self-transcendence: Deductive reformulation using developmental theories. *Advanced Nursing Science, 13*(4), 64–77.

Reed, P. G. (2008). Theory of self-transcendence. In M. J. Smith & P. R. Liehr (Eds.), *Middle range theory for nursing* (2nd ed., pp. 163–200). New York, NY: Springer Publishing.

Swanson, K. M. (1993). Nursing as informed caring for the well-being of others. *Journal of Nursing Scholarship, 25*(4), 352–357.

CHAPTER 13

Importance of Advocacy

Nurses are in the unique position of possessing the greatest amount of time to interact with the dying and their families. They can provide consistent holistic support; identify effective methods for communicating; anticipate needs; establish, confirm, and promote goals of care; ensure personalized care decisions are based on complete and accurate information; and assist in the fulfillment of desired means to achieve closure.

Advocacy is commonly proactive and requires effective communication skills. The nurse becomes aware of an issue of concern to be addressed and seeks resolution based on the best interest of the person being cared for and his or her family. This needs to occur before the issue or concern negatively affects the dying experience. Most issues involve improving symptom management, completion of unfinished business, and the promotion of the dignity and self-worth of the individual, thus encouraging transcendence toward a more accepting and prepared death.

The greatest barrier to achieving true advocacy for individuals under the care of the bedside nurse is the bedside nurse. Nurses continue to believe or buy into the subservient role assigned to them over the years, and express fears of "overstepping their boundaries," angering physicians, being accused of practicing medicine without a license or, the most devastating to our profession, just not wanting to take the time to get involved. The days of a nurse just coming to work to earn a paycheck and getting home as quickly as possible can no longer continue. Nurses must view their job as a knowledgeable and honored profession involved in an equal partnership with other medical professionals. There is much that nurses can contribute, and nurses are deserving of respect from the entire health care team.

Individuals under a nurse's care are often desperate for a voice and this voice must come from the nurse. The change in practice to embrace advocacy will be challenging for many nurses who already feel over-whelmed by assignments, documentation requirements, and manda-tory in-services. Adding the increased work of being an advocate can be viewed as almost impossible given the additional time required to make the extra phone calls and arrangements. Having been a nurse for over 30 years, I share this concern, but I have found that once you have made a positive difference for a grieving family, had a dying patient whisper thank you, or brought a smile to a dying person's once flat and emotion-less face, you will be hooked.

I am reminded of an expression that I will paraphrase: If you want to teach people how to build a ship, don't just focus on the necessary techni-cal skills, help them learn to love the sea and desire, above all else, to learn to sail. Nurses must be made aware of the difference they can make for the dying and their families when they act as their advocate. Finding the time to be advocates will never be easy, but the rewards are great and will nour-ish them as professionals and as human beings.

Acting as an advocate for the dying and their families requires strong communication skills. A nurse cannot address a concern if a discussion or an assessment does not take place. Often the dying and their families do not want to bother the nurse with a problem or concern. And, just as often, nurses may be aware of a concern, but since no one chooses to discuss it with them, they choose to ignore it. The nurse is glad for one less task and moves on quickly to another more pressing matter. This is an example of the classic "elephant in the room."

It is a very human response to ignore the uncomfortable with the hope it will just go away. Often an amazing personal and professional growth opportunity will be missed, especially when caring for the dying. I have chosen to view the "elephant in the room" as a friendly, sweet, and loving stuffed animal that makes me laugh and quiets any fears or frustrations about addressing the concern it represents. I cannot take full credit for this technique as I learned about it in a communication lecture through the End-of-Life National Education Consortium (ELNEC), but I do think I have allowed the original idea to evolve a bit farther. My elephant in the room is a large gray stuffed one that wears SpongeBob pajamas and black high-top tennis shoes. How could anyone ignore or fear such a cuddly creature?

When I am confronted with uncomfortable questions or difficult situ-ations that need to be discussed, I identify the scenario as the "elephant in the room." As soon as I make this mental connection, I am drawn to think about my SpongeBob-dressed friend and I smile to myself, take a deep breath, and address the situation. I have never regretted using this technique. Although some discussions were uncomfortable at first, they yielded great results. I was able to confirm terminal diagnosis, help establish goals of care, arrange early Christmases, and resolve many miscommunications.

A strong advocate never avoids the elephant in the room; instead he or she walks directly up to it and gives it a big hug. The avoidance of an opportunity to make a difference for a dying individual and his or her family could impact his or her ability to achieve a peaceful death. The missed opportunity can be a regret that will follow the nurse for the rest of his or her career; this is by far too great a consequence.

When a nurse assumes the role of advocate and addresses the elephant in the room, he or she is often confronted with various needs and requests that ultimately will provide holistic support. Orders may be needed to increase pain medication, decrease anxiety, reduce confusion, or provide some emotional comfort. The most common resolution is the placement of a call to the attending physician. The nurse must remember that he or she is acting in the best interest of the person under his or her care and no one should ever find fault with these efforts. The request can be phrased as, "Mrs. D is requesting. . . " and then provide justification for the request. It is also helpful to suggest a resolution, especially if the physician you are interacting with does not know the individual under your care. Consider the physician you are dealing with and know that timing is everything. A call placed at 3 A.M. is never appropriate if it can be addressed later in the day.

UNDERSTANDING AVAILABLE RESOURCES

The nurse must know his or her resources and seek other health care personnel involvement as needed. I recall caring for an elderly man dying of end-stage heart disease who was obviously depressed and frequently tearful. When I asked if there was anything I could do to help cheer him up, he would mumble something softly that I could barely hear. I could have walked away and dismissed the mumbling as confusion, but I knew in my heart he needed something. I chose to ask the family if they had any thoughts why Mr. R was so sad. They felt the sadness was due to the fact that Mr. R had not seen his dog Morgan for nearly 6 months.

I had to work with infectious disease staff, hospital administration, and the manager of the nursing unit for permission to allow Morgan to visit. The family had to ensure Morgan would be bathed and that all of his vaccinations were current. I had the family sign a contract agreeing to keep Morgan in Mr. R's room only, and to remove Morgan from the hospital if any staff, patients, or visitors complained about the noise he was making.

Finally, all approvals were obtained and Morgan was brought in for a visit. It was one of the most touching moments of my career when Morgan entered Mr. R's room. The dog instinctively knew to be quiet and walked quickly to Mr. R's bed. He saw he was asleep and climbed up on the bed, curled up next to Mr. R, and gently placed his head on Mr. R's chest. Mr. R never opened his eyes, but slowly moved his right arm to pet the dog's head. A smile soon spread across Mr. R's face that changed his features completely. The family and I became teary eyed as we watched this deep demonstration of love. To this day, I am happy for taking the time to bring a smile to Mr. R's face who died peacefully 3 days later.

SUPPORT OF CULTURE AND COMMUNICATION PREFERENCES

Being a good patient advocate can also include supporting cultural wishes and honoring established family communication preferences. This is again accomplished through effective communication. In the case of Mrs. P, I became aware of the intense sadness and grief the family was experiencing as they quietly sat by the bedside. It would have been easy to ignore, but I smiled to myself about confronting my elephant in the room, and decided to check further into my assessment. I asked the family if they could do one thing to celebrate the life of Mrs. P, what would it be?

I was told how much Mrs. P loved Christmas and how sad the family was at the thought they would never share another Christmas with her. This set in motion the plan for Christmas in July. Mrs. P's family demeanor changed dramatically as they began to plan a Christmas celebration. The quiet and sadness was replaced by stories of Mrs. P's Christmas extravagance and laughter. Even though Mrs. P rarely had the strength to open her eyes, you could sense her happiness. She would occasionally whisper a few words to her family that showed she approved of the plan, telling them where to find her recipes and where to buy certain food items.

After obtaining permission from the maintenance department for the lights and electrical decorations, permission from the unit manager to decorate, and promising the safety department all fire safety rules would be followed, the Christmas decorating began. It was not a difficult task to obtain permission and the way the project transformed the family made any inconvenience worth it.

The family transformed their grief into a celebration of Mrs. P's life. They got an emotional break that allowed them to share their love and to honor what Mrs. P meant to all of them. Soon there was Christmas music and wonderful smells of different foods. Mrs. P's room became the North Pole and her bed a mass of festive pillows and comforters. The activity also provided a much needed emotional break for the staff as they joined in by wearing the Santa hats brought in by the family. There truly was a transcendence that occurred from intense sadness and grief to a celebration of the life of Mrs. P.

As Mrs. P continued to decline, she spoke less to her family and seemed to be emotionally preparing to die. One evening I visited Mrs. P; her room was lit only by the Christmas tree lights and Christmas carols played softly in the background. Her family was asleep in nearby chairs and sofas, so I quietly sat down at Mrs. P's bedside. I held her hand and whispered how beautiful her room was and how grateful I was for the opportunity to help make her time here with us special. I told Mrs. P that I would continue to do everything in my power so she would not suffer and how lucky she was to have such a loving family. Mrs. P began to softly whisper something and I leaned in to hear. She was whispering that she loved me. Of course I immediately teared up, but somehow found the strength to tell her that I loved her, too.

Mrs. P died with her loving family around her. There were many tears, but there were smiles, too, knowing her death was so peaceful because she was surrounded by love and Christmas. I was not there when Mrs. P died. I was saddened by the news, but found comfort remembering her journey. It was such an honor to get to know this lovely lady and her family, and I will forever remember my small role in her peaceful death.

Being an advocate for individuals under our care is essential to helping provide for a peaceful death. Often the role can be emotionally painful when close relationships are formed, but I have found the sadness to be short lived as you become aware of the difference you make in another person's life. The memories the family will take with them will also help sustain them through their bereavement. Being an advocate should be viewed as an honor that allows a nurse to ensure all desired care is made possible.

A strong advocate provides closure and supports the grieving process as described with the interactions with Mrs. P. The role of advocate should also include clearly sharing established goals of care with other health care providers. This may require reminding physicians about patient wishes and reconfirming with family members about the choices they made.

It is essential, while in the role of advocate, that the nurse uses strong communication skills to educate the dying and their families through open discussions on risks versus benefits of treatments and care. Acting as an advocate allows the nurse to assist in the fulfillment of desired means to achieve closure. It can be a challenge addressing the elephant in the room but the mutual patient, family, and personal benefits are well worth the effort.

STEVEN'S PEACEFUL DEATH

The decision of the nurses caring for Steven to work with social work and to allow me to assist them is a basic role of being a patient advocate. The nurse needs to anticipate and assemble all support personnel, equipment, and medications necessary to provide for the identified care required to promote a peaceful death. Being a good advocate for Steven required making as much uninterrupted time as possible available for the parents to interact with their son, being present and reassuring, educating about differences in a normal dying process and suffering, and seeking the parents' input regarding care choices. Steven's parents needed some sense of control during this uncontrollable situation. This was provided by allowing them to dictate care choices and have direct involvement with Steven's care. Often being a good patient advocate requires knowing when you are not needed. Always clarify privacy needs. The need for privacy should never result in feelings of abandonment for the family. In Steven's case, the family asked for time alone because culturally they were a very private family. The nurse did not take this request personally and told the family she would remain available if they needed her.

CHAPTER 14

Achieving Compassionate Communication

Communication is one of the most essential skills required to provide quality evidence-based care for the dying and their families. It is impossible to convey compassion and caring without communicating. The ability for a dying individual and his or her family to know a nurse is genuine and caring is based on his or her ability to successfully communicate through touch, direct eye contact, use of a soft comforting voice, and positioning and posturing that is welcomed into an individual's personal space.

NONVERBAL AND VERBAL COMMUNICATION

Not all methods of nonverbal communication are universal and can be interpreted differently because of cultural influences. When the spoken word is not synchronized with nonverbal behavior, the message attempted to be communicated can be misinterpreted and result in negative interpretations. An example would be the nurse who states she was concerned how the individual under her care slept, but never stops looking at her clipboard. No eye contact is attempted. No nonverbal behaviors of concern, such as touching the hand or sitting down to await an answer. The message projected is one of indifference and lacks a true caring focus.

Communication impacts nursing care and the ability of a dying individual to feel comforted, respected, and listened to. The presence of these feelings promotes and supports essential emotions to sustain hope and to transcend fears of the dying process. An individual must know he or she is valued and viewed as a unique and special human being who deserves respect, and whose dignity will be honored and preserved.

The nonverbal behaviors of the nurse to promote these positive feelings can be as simple as placing a cool washcloth on the forehead of a dying individual, offering a cup of tea to a family member, or sitting in silence and actively listening to an individual's fears and concerns about dying. We cannot not communicate. Compassionate, nurturing behavior is predominately nonverbal as is more than 80% of all communication. Dying individuals and their families need nurses to convey their humanity and accessibility to gain their trust and be comforted during their final journey. Nurses must be aware of their nonverbal actions and know that the individuals they care for and their families are aware of how busy nurses are, so any extra time spent on comforting them will be deeply appreciated and will contribute greatly to their need to feel valued and safe.

CONVERSATIONS INITIATED BY THE DYING

Another method to help the dying and their families feel valued and respected is for conversations and open discussions initiated by the dying not to be ignored. Nurses are in the best position to pick up on the questions and concerns of the dying. Nurses are often the ones to identify the elephant in the room that is emphasized by the unspoken needs of individuals to obtain answers, to understand what is happening to them, and to express their wishes for care. This desire is often thwarted because of a nurse's failure to pick up on cues, or his or her desire to avoid an uncomfortable conversation.

The uncomfortable conversation that needs to occur often defines "the elephant in the room." Both parties know the role they need to play but choose to avoid because of fears of upsetting each other, overstepping authority, being so uncomfortable they cannot bear to take part in the discussion, or out of fear of providing/giving an answer that will confirm another's fears. Often, it is the health care provider's own sense of inadequacy or fear about death that prevents important discussions from occurring.

Nurses are trained to always refer back to the physician when an individual under his or her care has questions about the treatment or disease. It is important the nurse works in unison with the physician and supports the identified plan of care. The role of advocate would need to be addressed as part of supporting the family when they have questions or express wishes the physician does not address or chooses to ignore.

Avery Weisman (1972) described this desire to seek information about one's terminal state as a condition of lonely apprehension. DeSpelder and Strickland (2015) noted surveys that indicated the majority of individuals wanted to be told about their terminal illness. Health care providers must supply this information in a manner that reflects the individual's specific personality, familial, sociocultural, emotional, and stress-adaptive resources. Often, health care providers will avoid initiating these conversations because of concerns over diminishing the terminally ill individual's ability to cope. They will rationalize delaying providing important information until the individual asks specific questions. The underlying motivation of the health care provider in this instance is often that of avoidance. Conversations that entail a poor or terminal prognosis often emphasize health care provider feelings of failure and/or increase personal awareness of one's own mortality. This overidentification with the dying can result in additional barriers to communication. The avoidance of important discussions is yet another example of the elephant in the room that must be addressed.

> Communicating a diagnosis is a crucial event in patient care. How it is done can influence a patient's attitude toward the illness, response to treatment, and ability to cope. The content of such a conversation depends on a number of factors, including the doctor's preferences for breaking bad news, the patient's receptivity to the facts, and the expected prognosis. (DeSpelder & Strickland, 2015, p. 182)

BREAKING BAD NEWS

Breaking bad news requires a series of discussions to relay all needed information. It is not unusual that the initial shock of receiving negative news results in fragmented comprehension of information. Care providers can improve upon their initial and future discussions regarding an individual's terminal illness by following Ken Doka's (2009) eight principles for delivering bad news.

1. Keep it simple
2. Ask yourself, "What does the diagnosis mean to the patient?"
3. Meet on "cool ground" first; get to know the patient before presenting the news
4. Wait for questions
5. Do not argue with denial
6. Ask questions yourself
7. Do not destroy all hope
8. Do not say anything that is not true (pp. 35–36)

The incorporation of the PEWTER (prepare, evaluate, warning, telling, emotional response, and regrouping) method for delivering bad news can further refine Doka's (2009) communication technique for delivering bad news (Keefe-Cooperman & Brady-Amoon, 2013). The resulting consolidation of suggested principles for effective communication is as follows:

1. **Preparing:** This component includes the establishment of rapport prior to counseling, and arranging to have discussions in a quiet, private, and supportive location.

2. **Evaluation:** This component encompasses a review of what the individual to be counseled desires to know, already knows, and what the new information to be provided could potentially mean to them.

3. **Warning:** This component is essential to the delivery of communicating bad news. The individual being counseled often requires advance notice to emotionally prepare to receive information that will be negative in nature. This component of breaking bad news is often referred to as a "warning shot." A warning shot helps to prepare the individual being counseled that the information to be provided will be personally upsetting early in the conversation, can reduce the emotional shock that can accompany receiving bad news, and can allow for an increased comprehension of the information provided.

4. **Telling:** This component includes a conscious effort to supply all information in honest, open, and easily understood language; and provides time for the individual to absorb the information. The time needed to comprehend the information provided must be established by the individual being counseled and involves the caregiver sitting in silence until the conversation is reinitiated by the individual.

5. **Emotional response:** This component is an extension of the telling phase of delivering bad news. It includes waiting for questions, not arguing with denial, providing nonverbal gestures of emotional support such as holding the individual's hand, placing a hand on the shoulder, and allowing for varied demonstrations of emotion to occur without interruption such as crying, swearing, or pacing.

6. **Regrouping:** This component requires the asking of questions by the caregiver, reframing to promote a new focus for hope, remaining truthful, and introducing the need to reestablish/confirm goals of care.

Communicating bad news is not the only form of communication needed when caring for the dying and their families. Communication skills must be learned, and the most important use of good communication skills is essential to the role of advocate. The wishes and personal goals of the dying must be honored, respected, and clearly understood by all care providers.

A good communicator must first be a good listener and a good observer. As stated earlier, most communication is nonverbal, so the caregiver must possess the ability to discern physical cues such as the presence of eye contact, facial expressions, and body gestures. None of this is possible if a care provider is focused on his or her own agenda and only asking questions that limit responses and feed into an individual's hesitancy to challenge his or her doctors. Communication is considered "the single most valuable asset of the skilled doctor" (DeSpelder & Strickland, 2015, p. 184).

The dying patient's desire to talk about death can be greatly hindered if the health care provider utilizes some of the most common communication barriers identified by DeSpelder and Strickland (2015), which include false reassurance of health, denial of pending-death fears, changing of the subject to a more cheerful topic or in an attempt to distract the dying individual, use of fatalism to inappropriately reduce or minimize fears, and redirection to identify an alternate focus for the individual's question away from death. These responses have their foundation in the discomfort caregivers experience when they must acknowledge they cannot rescue or cure a dying patient (Stanton-Chapple, 2010).

Effective communication can promote hope through the establishment of a positive attitude and resultant outcome. The creation of a positive atmosphere can promote psychosocial healing regardless of the prognosis. If a negative atmosphere is allowed to continue, it can result in the development of a negative focus with associated despondency and despair (DeSpelder & Strickland, 2015).

THE COMFORT NURSING INITIATIVE

Another method to improve communication was developed by Wittenberg-Lyles, Goldsmith, Ferrell, and Reagan (2013) called the COMFORT nursing initiative. It was designed to specifically address the need to Communicate, use Orientation and opportunity, acknowledge the need for Mindful presence, emphasize the role of the Family, recognize and effectively utilize communication Openings, support the need for Relating to the individual and his or her family, and to address the essential role of a Team approach to enhance and promote effective communication.

The COMFORT nursing initiative identifies the ability to communicate as a necessary skill that requires learning and practice to effectively bear witness to the suffering of an individual, provide and receive person-centered focused messages both verbally and nonverbally, and address the unique holistic communication needs of the terminally ill. The essential use of verbal clarity and nonverbal behaviors that encourage eye contact, supportive posturing, nodding in agreement, and the avoidance of fidgeting on the part of the health care provider. The focus is on delivering patient-centered compassionate care that meets the needs of the individual and his or her family.

The recognition of orientation and opportunity identifies the need to communicate within the understanding and literacy levels of the individual, acknowledge possible vulnerability due to inadequate information and education, identify and support cultural issues and humility, and develop a plan for addressing specific communication and care needs utilizing strategies unique to the individual's cognitive and emotional capacities that promotes an awareness and an increased likelihood of understanding of prognosis and care options. The opportunity to provide education is encouraged in an effort to ensure informed care decisions.

Mindful presence is essential as it emphasizes the use of empathy, active listening, demonstrates an understanding of cultural humility, employs effective nonverbal communication techniques, and acknowledges the nonverbal cues of the individual receiving care. Wittenberg-Lyles et al. (2010) emphasized mindful self-monitoring for the care provider to encourage openness to more than one perspective and to promote curiosity and attentiveness. The need for the health care provider to pass judgment is discouraged and the ability to quickly adapt to unique interaction situations is encouraged.

The incorporation of family into methods of effective communication identified the important role of family, their unique communication patterns, and encouraged the identification of varying family caregiver requirements. The unit of care for a terminally ill and dying individual must include his or her family, and there must be a commitment on the part of the health care provider to meet both their needs. One cannot separate the cultural and psychosocial effects of family on an individual. This deeply embedded influence can be effectively addressed to promote and support established goals of care and to honor the important role family has in the life and care of the individual.

Openings speak to the impact of pivotal events that resulted in changes in family and individual care dynamics, the need to establish methods of communication that can overcome existing tensions, and the identification of methods to more effectively provide disclosure. The opportunity for caregivers to introduce change and promote new methods of coping must be identified and effectively utilized to assist the individual and his or her family to adapt to the many changes they will encounter in the dying process. Openings encourage health care providers to remain vigilant and not ignore the opportunities to assist successful adaptation to possible painful change. These opportunities often occur early when discussions are held regarding diagnosis, treatment decisions, and disease progression.

Relating embraces and supports the multiple care goals of the individual and the family and not those of the health care provider. It accepts the presence of conflicting goals, and the need to utilize effective communication to identify "common ground" to allow for the development of mutually accepted goals of care. Care providers must be willing to meet and work with individuals and their families at their current levels of understanding and acceptance of the disease process. Frequent retelling of information may occur as all parties involved attempt to absorb information and address the impact this information will have on their lives. Empathy and compassion are essential as short-term memory becomes limited due to the extensive stress encountered while trying to process the dramatic changes occurring for the individual. Bad news can only be digested in small doses and the caregiver should be prepared to provide multiple interactions at the unique pace and frequency set by the individual. Health care providers must function within the unique values and perspectives established by the dying patient and his or her family and not by their own agenda.

The final component of the COMFORT nursing initiative is the utilization of a team. The importance of interdisciplinary teamwork is emphasized as essential to promote successful collaboration to address established goals of care. The sharing of observations and recommendations of specialists in their field is a proven strategy utilized within palliative care to provide individualized support for the dying and their families. Communication required to effectively share common goals and to focus on quality end-of-life care is practiced and utilized extensively as all members of the team work to remain "on the same page." It is also recognized and accepted that no single individual can provide all necessary care and support. The utilization of professionals with the same focus to support the goals of a dying individual and his or her family remains the most efficient method to provide individualized holistic symptom management for the dying and his or her family.

In summary, the COMFORT nursing initiative addresses a method of communication when interacting with the terminally ill. It recommends:

- **Communicate:** Get to know the patient's story and the family. Establish a rapport.
- **Orientation and opportunity:** Identify understanding of illness, utilize concepts of cultural humility. Get to know family values and how they interact.
- **Mindfulness:** Make good observations and do not interject own values.
- **Family:** Include family in discussions and be aware of their impact on supporting the patient.
- **Openings:** Have goals of care focused conversations. Utilize opportunities to explore and clarify needs.
- **Relating:** Sharing one's self and using self-disclosure to establish trust. Share stories of personal experiences with patients and families to demonstrate understanding.
- **Team:** Effective communication will require the assistance of other palliative team members to help clarify and support the desires/wishes identified by the patient and family.

This chapter on communication cannot begin to address the extensive information available to health care providers to improve their ability to effectively communicate. A belief exists that good communicators are born with their ability. This is not true. Individuals may have a heightened ability to pick up nonverbal cues, changes in voice patterns, and posturing. There may be an increased ability to empathize or to discern others' emotions, but the ability to communicate effectively is learned. It requires practice and self-awareness. The need to pursue professional and personal agendas must be abandoned and the use of an open and accepting focus to truly hear what an individual is expressing is essential. The ability to quiet our minds, let go of personal agendas, be fully present, and therapeutically listen can only occur with education, practice, and dedication. The ability to effectively communicate is the greatest gift we can give to our dying patients and their families, and it is the most important skill health care providers can possess.

The communication skills provided in this chapter were never given an important emphasis in this author's nursing education. The hope was to provide a chapter that emphasized the difference a nurse can make if a commitment is made to becoming a skilled and effective communicator. It is impossible to become a strong advocate for individuals under your care without strong communication skills.

The ability to effectively communicate is essential to all sections of the CARES tool. Verbal and nonverbal cues are needed to fully assess successful symptom management. Health care providers must be aware of the numerous factors that influence individuals' ability to communicate their symptom management and spiritual needs. Communication is influenced by cultural and family influences; fears of addiction, weakness, and unworthiness; and decisions to remain stoic, to not "bother" the health care provider, or to deny the symptoms because of the fear the disease is progressing.

The effects of culture should be emphasized. It is difficult to correctly anticipate an individual's reactions based solely on culture. It is common for an individual to be influenced not only by ethnic-based values but parental and societal values as well. It is important for the health care providers to effectively communicate with individuals under their care and identify the values and rituals desired to assist in adapting to the many stressors they will be confronted with during their end-of-life journey. (See suggested readings in Chapter 25 for additional resources on cultural influences on end-of-life care.)

Further education and training to improve the ability to effectively communicate is encouraged. This can be achieved by attending the End-of-Life Nursing Education Consortium (ELNEC) program and reviewing references focused on communication such as the Wittenberg-Lyles et al. (2013) work titled *Communication in Palliative Nursing*, and articles published on the COMFORT nursing initiative.

Applying the communication techniques discussed in this chapter to the sample case of Steven's end-of-life care discussed throughout the beginning of this book, one can easily see how essential communication was to providing the resources and support for Steven, his family, and the nurses providing care. Based on the components of the COMFORT nursing initiative, the following supportive end-of-life communication efforts were made.

Communicate: Steven's family was aware that Steven was actively dying. They were loving and attentive, and desperately wanted to be involved with ensuring Steven's comfort. In an effort to reduce anxiety, education was provided to help family members to differentiate between a normal dying process and suffering.

Orientation and opportunity: Steven's parents were tearful and sat close to the bedside. Their faces showed concern and they appeared anxious. Education was the focus of much of the interaction as attempts were made to address their primarily nonverbal behavior and encourage questions.

Mindfulness: The family was informed of my availability and much time was spent sitting with them in supportive silence in an effort to reassure and provide a therapeutic presence.

Family: Steven was incapable of any social or purposeful interaction. His family was acting in his best interest. The goals of care were to keep Steven comfortable so he could die peacefully with his family at his side. The family requested to be allowed some privacy to experience Steven's final moments. Their request was honored and the health care staff remained available for any questions or concerns. It was difficult to not be directly involved and provide a supportive presence during the last moments of Steven's life, but it was equally important to honor the family's request for privacy.

Openings: The family's nonverbal behavior meanings were clarified and education on the normal dying process was provided along with options to reduce the BiPAP that was causing involuntary heaving-like chest arching respirations as it forced air into Steven's lungs. Open-ended questions were used to assess for any further education and support needs.

Relating: The family made it clear they were very private and were prepared to address their son's death alone. They confirmed they felt well supported and now wanted to focus on the last few moments they had with their son. All interruptions were carefully screened and the family was placed in control of all activities to support their request and to demonstrate the understanding of their wishes by the health care team. They were aware of our availability if needed.

Team: The social worker, chaplain, and unit nurses remained available for any questions or concerns. It was made clear to the family that I (palliative care NP) was acting on behalf of the primary physician who remained available by phone. Frequent visual assessments were made of the family to identify any issues or concerns. Most of my work during the final moments of Steven's life centered on the nursing staff's professional grief. They expressed frustration about not being able to help. This concern was reframed to recognize the important role they played as advocate, the value of their therapeutic presence, and the support they were providing the family to allow them the privacy they desired.

REFERENCES

DeSpelder, L. A., & Strickland, A. L. (2015). *The last dance: Encountering death and dying* (10th ed.). New York, NY: McGraw-Hill.

Doka, K. J. (2009). *Counseling individuals with life threatening illness.* New York, NY: Springer Publishing.

Keefe-Cooperman, K., & Brady-Amoon, P. (2013). Breaking bad news in counseling: Applying the PEWTER model in the school setting. *Journal of Creativity in Mental Health, 8*(3), 265–277.

Stanton-Chapple, H. (2010). *No place for dying: Hospitals and the ideology of rescue.* Walnut Creek, CA: Left Coast Press.

Weisman, A. D. (1972). *On dying and denying: A psychiatric study of terminality.* New York, NY: Behavioral Publications.

Wittenberg-Lyles, E., Goldsmith, J., Ferrell, B., & Ragan, S. (2013). *Communication in palliative nursing.* New York, NY: Oxford University Press.

CHAPTER 15

Promoting a Peaceful Death

Apeaceful death can only truly be defined by the individual. For many, a peaceful death is one that occurs without pain or suffering. A sense of peace can be achieved when the dying are able to transcend their fears and accept whatever is to come beyond their earthly existence. As discussed in other chapters, transcendence is only possible when physical symptoms are controlled so the individual can focus his or her limited energy on accepting their final journey.

Ideally, a peaceful death would include closure. The opportunity to say good-bye, apologize, forgive, and reaffirm love for family members and special persons in the life of the dying is one form of closure. Others include completing unfinished business, instructing family members on business transactions, and making wishes known for the dispersing of personal belongings.

Legacy work can also add to successful closure. The dying are made aware of their valuable contributions to their families and to society. There are many creative methods to memorialize an individual from handprint pillows, memory quilts, journals, videos, and jewelry. All are designed to share a part of the dying individual's life and to promote the development of comforting memories.

One of the worst forms of suffering is to die without feeling your life had meaning, feeling you did nothing to improve the world, and knowing there will be no one to grieve for you. Affirmations of love and leaving a legacy through children and grandchildren often provide the self-worth necessary to accept death and the losses it entails for most individuals.

As death approaches the overall fatigue and loss of ability to fight helps to enhance acceptance. For some this does not occur and the very terror of dying can cause extensive emotional and spiritual pain. Some of this suffering can be minimized by religious rituals such as receiving the last rites as provided for those of the Catholic faith, but others cannot be comforted and may require sedation to endure their final hours of life.

Anxiety over death and dying becomes more prevalent in the aging population. Confronting mortality at any age is a struggle, but for the 65+ age group it can cause many individuals to experience severe anxiety and depression as they encounter increased losses in the form of friends, family, self-worth, dignity, and personal identity (Edmondson, Park, Chaudoir, & Wortmann, 2008). Nichols (2010) noted "People fear death because they have no positive vision of afterlife" (p. 33). Edmondson et al. (2008) noted a strong relationship between spiritual beliefs such as a belief in an afterlife, and emotional, psychological, and religious comfort. Literature provides evidence that spirituality is central to the dying person (Edmondson et al., 2008, 2010). It is becoming more apparent that care of the dying is much more than just care of the body. To help facilitate a peaceful death, health care providers must learn to care for the soul (Puchalski & Ferrell, 2010). This will require an emphasis on cultivating warm and accepting relationships with dying patients and families, developing extraordinary listening and communication skills, and striving to remove fears of abandonment and worthlessness (Puchalski & Ferrell, 2010). Caring for the soul means ". . . recognizing the power in our own humanity to make a difference in the lives of others and valuing it as highly as our expertise" (Puchalski & Ferrell, 2010, p. xx).

Unresolved questions and fears about the existence of an afterlife, heaven, eternal damnation, and ceasing to exist can become dominant concerns for the dying (Nichols, 2010). Comfort care becomes enmeshed in the highly religious and philosophical realms of the human need for assurances of life significance and worthiness of an afterlife (Edmondson et al., 2008; Yalom, 2009).

THE ROLE OF THE HEALTH CARE PROVIDER IN PROMOTING A PEACEFUL DEATH

Often, health care providers can assist with these needed assurances simply by being fully present and listening to the dying as they attempt to organize their thoughts and challenge their fears (City of Hope & AACN, 2012; Puchalski & Ferrell, 2010). Frequently health care providers may struggle with their own perceptions of what occurs after death and are challenged to remain in a supportive, noncommitted, listening role. Taking the time to truly listen to a patient without judgment could prove to be one of the most valuable practices health care providers can provide individuals under their care, their families, and themselves. The very presence of a health care provider willing to take the time to listen and share in the emotional and spiritual journey of the dying process signifies respect and acknowledges the value of the patient and his or her family (City of Hope & AACN, 2012; Nichols, 2010; Puchalski & Ferrell, 2010). This time is actually the most sacred for the nurturing of the spirit, the soul, the very essence of the individual now confronting their mortality (Edmondson et al., 2008; Nichols, 2010).

The communication techniques of listening, silence, and providing an atmosphere of total acceptance can often provide more physical relief for a terminally ill patient than any sedative or narcotic (City of Hope & AACN, 2012; Puchalski & Ferrell, 2010). Yalom (2009) stated that, "One can offer no greater service to someone facing death than to offer him or her your sheer presence" (p. 125). Just being present is an affirmation to the dying and their families that they will never be abandoned. It is the human connection that is important. Health care providers need to achieve closeness, communicate from the heart, and risk confronting one's own fears of mortality. The dying often have so much they need to share, and so much they can teach if we could learn to listen with our hearts and ignore the cold logic our brains tempt us to interject (Wise, 2007; Yalom, 2009).

Religiosity and spirituality can offer answers to questions about dying and an afterlife. Dezutter et al. (2009) noted spiritual beliefs ". . . provide individuals with a sense of predictability and control that may protect against overwhelming anxiety provoked by the perspective of death" (p. 74). Emotional and spiritual support is essential when caring for the terminally ill and family (American Medical Association, 2012; Byock, Twohig, Merriman, & Collins, 2006; City of Hope & AACN, 2012; Douglas, Murtagh, Chambers, Howse, & Ellershaw, 2009; Ferrell & Coyle, 2010). The End-of-Life Nursing Education Consortium (ELNEC) project developed by the City of Hope and AACN (2012) identified specific psychological and spiritual needs of the dying and their families requiring physical, emotional, and educational support from the nurse. Addressing fears of the dying process, abandonment, the unknown, identifying signs and symptoms of nearing death versus suffering, helping families understand the role of emotional withdrawal by the patient in the active dying process, and the continued need for touch and presence are common teaching points. A strong religious belief in the afterlife can reduce many of the fears of the unknown and of immortality helping to reduce possible death anxiety (Edmondson et al., 2008; Nichols, 2010).

Dezutter et al. (2009) cited Jung's observation that all major world religions have a system or process they use to prepare for death. Jung noted that often the second half of life's primary goal is to prepare for death. Religions provide meaning to the process of dying. Spiritual beliefs are considered ". . . the most important and effective way to put death into perspective and to find meaning in life" (p. 74).

The desire to cure and/or correct problems in an attempt to avoid death remains a focus for many health care providers (Puchalski & Ferrell, 2010). A dying person does not necessarily require further "fixing." Puchalski and Ferrell (2010) noted a healing of the spirit can occur during the dying process allowing individuals and their families to find ". . . meaning and hope even in the midst of dying" (p. 12). "Fixing" can lead to hopelessness, emotional suffering, and frustration because of existing medical limitations and the narrow definitions of success. Spiritual healing can continue to occur on many levels and provide renewed meaning and hope for the dying (McClain-Jacobson et al., 2004; Puchalski & Ferrell, 2010).

Training nurses to provide effective care to patients and family members during the dying process is an important skill to learn as part of nursing practice (Byock, 2012; City of Hope & AACN, 2012; Parish et al., 2006). There is a continual need for emotional and physical support, reinforcement of the decision process, and acknowledgement of the grieving process by nursing and medical staff (Catlin & Carter, 2002). Any sense of abandonment can be emotionally devastating to patients and families in the dying process (City of Hope & AACN, 2012; Ferrell & Coyle, 2010; Quill, 1996). Clear and open communication with health care professionals is essential. The need becomes more urgent with the family's awareness of approaching death (Byock, 2012; Parish et al., 2006). Issues of perceived suffering should be addressed and readdressed to help comfort the family and assist coping as they witness the death of the loved one and work through the grieving process (Brajtman, 2005).

SUPPORTING THE DYING PERSON'S SENSE OF SPIRITUALITY

There is minimal research on the role the belief in an afterlife plays on coping with the dying process. Much of the research was completed with healthy college students resulting in questions of ecological validity and generalizability (McClain-Jacobson et al., 2004). The concept of achieving spiritual well-being seems to transcend religious barriers and provides a broader focus to appeal to patients without traditional religious convictions (2004). It promotes a shift beyond just the religious. Puchalski and Ferrell (2010) defined spirituality as:

> . . . a term that refers to many dimensions of a person's life. It has been described as the essence of humanity by Frankl in 1963, and how people find a sense of who they are or their personhood. Spirituality can also be understood as one's relationship to a transcendence that for some people might be God and for others might be different concepts of how they see themselves in the world and in relationships outside themselves. (p. 21)

A dying individual's sense of spirituality must be understood and supported if health care professionals are to assist him or her in achieving spiritual well-being. The dying need to transcend the commonplace and arrive at what they define as meaningful to them, and drawing on past accomplishments such as those derived from legacy work can assist in this process. They must feel their lives have value, that they are loved and cherished, and possess a strong sense of who they really are to access the deeper meanings of life within their soul. The dyings' spirituality is essential for transcendence as they search for meaning and the sacred or holy, whether religious in focus or not (Puchalski & Ferrell, 2010).

The act of dying peacefully and well supported is a complicated and highly technical process requiring focused education and training for health care providers. The attainment of spiritual well-being is an important component to achieving a peaceful death. There is a need for engaged and attentive health care providers willing to take the time to listen and share in the emotional and spiritual journey of the dying. Health care personnel play an important role in acknowledging and preserving the dignity and self-worth of a dying individual essential to the achievement of spiritual well-being.

It is important to note that the dying are not broken as much as they are following a normal life course. The health care provider must remember there is always a possibility for some level of emotional, spiritual, and/or psychological healing that can occur during the dying process. Dying is truly much more than just care of the body; health care professionals must also care for the soul. There is a need to provide spiritual and religious support for the terminally ill as they face their fears and beliefs about dying and struggle to achieve spiritual well-being as they define it. If the dying and their families can have their spiritual issues effectively identified and supported, the possibility for a peaceful death increases.

Cultural, race, religious, and lifestyle norms may be in conflict with the final spiritual need to come to terms with the existence of an afterlife. Communication is essential. Spiritual, cultural, and psychosocial support becomes challenging when the values of the health care provider are in direct conflict with the dying elderly patient. Unconditional support must be provided (Byock, 2012). An ethics consult, spiritual counselors, and social workers should be available for both grieving families and staff (American Medical Association, 2012; City of Hope & AACN, 2012; Frommelt, 1991).

The need to provide evidence-based end-of-life care is well established in literature. Issues addressing beliefs and fears of dying, the attainment of spiritual well-being, and promoting a peaceful death continue to go unrecognized in many institutions. The hospice and palliative care strategy to treat the entire person has helped to address some of these issues. Spiritual beliefs have evolved to mean so much more than just religious conviction

(Ferrell & Coyle, 2010). Puchalski and Ferrell (2010) provided a definition developed by an interdisciplinary group attending a spirituality consensus conference in February 2009.

> Spirituality is the aspect of humanity that refers to the way individuals seek and express meaning and purpose, and the way they experience their connectedness to the moment, to self, to others, to nature, and to the significant or sacred. (p. 25)

Hospitals must continue to develop programs that address the spiritual needs of the dying and their families as they define them, and better prepare health care providers for the associated issues they will confront as our population continues to age. Dying is an undeniable fact of life. Health care providers must become experts in the medical aspects of caring for the dying, but they must also be prepared to address the spiritual aspects of caring for the soul (Byock et al., 2006; City of Hope & AACN, 2012; Puchalski & Ferrell, 2010; Yalom, 2009).

A patient's spirituality must be understood and supported by health care professionals. It is the very essence of who the patient is as a human being. It encompasses uniqueness and should be celebrated. The dyings' spiritual well-being is dependent upon a sense of self-worth, dignity, and personal identity. Knowing they will not be forgotten and their life was meaningful are essential components of spiritual well-being. A strong sense of self is a requirement for achieving spiritual well-being and ultimately a peaceful death. The literature reaffirmed health care providers' important role in promoting and nurturing spiritual well-being through actively listening to the needs and concerns of a dying patient, and just being present. Presence without an associated task demonstrates unquestioning support and respect, and is one of the most challenging acts for a task-oriented nurse to accomplish. The humanity of the health care provider was acknowledged as the most important variable required to assist in the development of a dying patient's sense of spiritual well-being. Humanity was valued over any medication or procedure.

A sense of spiritual well-being is important to everyone as it requires feelings of worthiness, value, and a sense of purpose to flourish. This concept embraces an even greater importance for the dying. A strong sense of spiritual well-being provides the emotional strength and courage to confront issues of an afterlife. Persons with a strong religious focus often take comfort in the anticipation of heaven or seeing loved ones. The nonreligious-focused patient takes comfort in knowing he or she lived a life of value and worth, and will pass on a meaningful legacy to his or her family. Both views require a strong sense of spirituality fostered by the knowledge they are loved and their life had meaning. Ultimately, the literature review equated the promoting and nurturing of spiritual well-being as actually caring for the soul.

In the Foreword for Puchalski and Ferrell's (2010) *Making Health Care Whole: Integrating Spirituality into Patient Care*, Dr. Rachel Naomi Remen summarized the importance of caring for the soul in this excerpt.

Caring for the soul requires that we be fully present in situations we cannot control and patient as a genuine meaning and a direction unfold. It means seeing familiar things in new ways, listening rather than speaking, learning from patients rather than teaching them, and cultivating the capacity to be amazed. It means recognizing the power in your own humanity to make a difference in the lives of others and valuing it as highly as our expertise. Finally, it means discovering that healthcare is a front-row seat on mystery and sitting in that seat with open eyes. (p. xx)

REFERENCES

American Medical Association. (2012). *The EPEC (Education in Palliative and End of Life Care) project*. Retrieved from http://www.epec.net/epec_core.php

Brajtman, S. (2005). Helping the family through the experience of terminal restlessness. *Journal of Hospice & Palliative Nursing, 7*(2), 73–81. Retrieved from HPNA database: http://www.hpna.org

Byock, I. (2012). *The best care possible* (pp. 52–90). Retrieved from http://www.amazon.com/s/ref=nb_sb_ss_i_8_8?url=search-alias%3Ddigital-text&field-keywords=the+best+care+possible&sprefix=The+best%2Cdigital-text%2C256

Byock, I., Twohig, J. S., Merriman, M., & Collins, K. (2006). Promoting excellence in end-of-life care: A report on innovative models of palliative care. *Journal of Palliative Medicine, 9*(1), 137–151.

Catlin, A., & Carter, B. (2002). State of the art. Creation of a neonatal end-of-life palliative care protocol. *Journal of Perinatology, 22*(3), 184–195. Retrieved from CINHAL database.

City of Hope, & AACN. (2012). Final hours of life. *End of Life Nursing Education Consortium*. Duarte, CA: ELNEC.

Dezutter, J., Soenens, B., Luyckx, K., Bruyneel, S., Vansteenkiste, M., Duriez, B., & Hutsebaut, D. (2009). The role of religion in death attitudes: Distinguishing between religious belief and style of processing religious contents. *Death Studies, 33,* 73–92.

Douglas, C., Murtagh, F. E. M., Chambers, E. J., Howse, M., & Ellershaw, J. (2009). Symptom management for the adult patient dying with advanced chronic kidney disease: A review of the literature and development of evidence-based guidelines by a United Kingdom expert consensus group. *Palliative Medicine, 23*(2), 103–110.

Edmondson, D., Park, C. L., Chaudoir, S. R., & Wortmann, J. H. (2008). Death without God: Religious struggle, death concerns, and depression in the terminally ill. *Psychology Science, 19*(8), 745–758.

Ferrell, B. R., & Coyle, N. (Eds.). (2010). *Oxford textbook of palliative nursing* (3rd ed.). New York, NY: Oxford University Press.

Frommelt, K. H. M. (1991). The effects of death education on nurses' attitudes toward caring for terminally ill persons and their families. *American Journal of Hospice & Palliative Care, 8*(5), 37–43.

McClain-Jacobson, C., Rosenfeld, B., Kosinski, A., Pessin, H., Cimino, J. E., & Breitbart, W. (2004). Belief in an afterlife, spiritual well-being and end-of-life despair in patients with advanced cancer. *General Hospital Psychiatry, 26*, 484–486.

Nichols, T. (2010). *Death and afterlife: A theological introduction*. [Electronic Version]. Grand Rapids, MI: Brazos Press. Accessed from Kindle Books at http://www.amazon.com/s/ref=nb_sb_ss_i_1_19?url=search-alias%3Ddigital-text&field-keywords=death+and+afterlife+a+theological+introduction&sprefix=Death+and+afterlife%2Cdigital-text%2C210

Parish, K., Glaetzer, K., Grbich, C., Hammond, L., Hegarty, M., & McHugh, A. (2006). Dying for attention: Palliative care in the acute setting. *Australian Journal of Advanced Nursing, 24*(2), 21–25. Retrieved from CINHAL database.

Puchalski, C. M., & Ferrell, B. R. (2010). *Making health care whole: Integrating spiritually into practice*. [Electronic edition]. West Conshohocken, PA: Templeton Press.

Quill, T. E. (1996). *A midwife through the dying process: Stories of healing and hard choices at the end of life*. Baltimore, MD: Johns Hopkins University Press.

Wise, R. L. (2007). *Crossing the threshold of eternity: What the dying can teach the living*. [Electronic Book-Kindle Version]. Ventura, CA: Regal Books. Retrieved from http://www.amazon.com/s/ref=nb_sb_noss_1?url=search-alias%3Ddigital-text&field-keywords=Crossing+the+threshold+of+eternity

Yalom, I. D. (2009). *Staring at the sun: Overcoming the terror of death*. San Francisco, CA: Josey-Bass.

CHAPTER 16

Case Studies

As health care providers, we have the special privilege to walk with others to the "edge of life." These words were stated during a palliative care conference many years ago and still resonate with many health care providers who have the privilege to care for the dying. This may seem a strange way to view care of the dying, but for many it is the caregiver who is truly blessed and will be forever changed by the experience.

The following is a case that was given alternate endings to demonstrate what can go right and what can go terribly wrong when caring for the dying. The use of the same scenario is intentional, so the differences in care can be more readily understood and the effective use of the CARES tool can be accentuated.

Mr. F was a 78-year-old gentleman with a history of uncontrolled type 1 diabetes, end-stage cardiomyopathy, and acute renal insufficiency. He was brought to the emergency room by his elderly friend because of generalized chest pain that he rated 5/10 and acute fatigue. Mr. F was short of breath (respirations 32), emaciated, pale, and diaphoretic, with a blood pressure of 82/40. An echocardiogram showed an enlarged heart, a near-total akinetic left ventricle, and an estimated ejection fraction of less than 5%.

Case #1: Mr. F agreed to a do not resuscitate (DNR) status and stated he knew he was dying. He was placed on a morphine patient-controlled analgesia (PCA) system at 1 mg/hr with as needed boluses of 0.5 mg every 15 minutes as needed and oxygen per nasal cannula at 2 L/min. Hospice was contacted and would be speaking to Mr. F in the morning. He was admitted to the medical unit with orders for comfort measures only.

Using the CARES tool as a guide, his nurse clarified what comfort measures meant to Mr. F and obtained the following orders and support:

> **Comfort:** Orders were obtained to stop all lab draws, reduce his IV to KVO, and have a diet as tolerated. Titration orders for the morphine PCA were clarified, confirming the plan to continue to titrate up to patient comfort.

Airway: The nurse was aware the morphine PCA would help Mr. F tolerate his increasing shortness of breath and planned to continue to titrate as needed. She elevated the head of Mr. F's bed to comfort, and noted increasing oral-pharyngeal secretions and requested an order for glycopyrrolate.

Restlessness: Mr. F. became very restless after the initial assessment but denied an increase in his pain. Bladder distention was noted by the nurse, and an order was obtained for an indwelling urinary catheter. Mr. F had an immediate output of 500 cc and was resting more comfortably. An order for haloperidol as needed was obtained in preparation of possible future restlessness and/or terminal delirium. The nurse lowered the lights in the room to maintain a calm and supportive environment.

Emotional support: Mr. F denied having any family and requested his friend be allowed to stay with him. The friend was visibly upset, and the nurse took the time to explain what was happening and to listen to the friend's concerns that Mr. F did not suffer. The friend was treated as a family member. He requested that they be allowed to watch a hunting show on television, as this was their favorite activity at home. The nurse positioned a chair next to Mr. F's bed and turned on the television. Mr. F continued to struggle to breathe but appeared peaceful with his friend at his side. The nurse checked on them frequently and made sure they were aware she was available if they needed her. The nurse sat with Mr. F when she noted his friend had fallen asleep. Mr. F talked softly about his life as the nurse held his hand. Mr. F closed his eyes and became unresponsive to the nurse's voice and touch. His respirations became more shallow and irregular with 30- to 45-second episodes of apnea, and the nurse noted increased oropharyngeal secretions and remedicated with glycopyrrolate. Mr. F. began to moan softly and had a distinct facial grimace. This was a change from the softened peaceful expression the nurse noted earlier. The nurse gave a 0.5 mg bolus of morphine through the PCA and after 15 minutes noted a return of a more peaceful expression on Mr. F's face. Mr. F continued to rest comfortably, but his apnea episodes increased over the next 3 hours. The nurse noted Mr. F's mottled feet and knees and generalized body coolness. She obtained a blood pressure of 50/palpitation. Mr. F's friend was at his side when he died peacefully a few hours later. The friend was supported by the nurse and pastoral care and assisted with funeral home arrangements.

Self-care: The nurse became tearful as she was touched by Mr. F's peacefulness and acceptance of his dying. She took pride in knowing she made his last few hours comfortable and supported his friend. She shared her story with the staff in morning report and was listened to and supported by her coworkers. Her manager brought her a cup of tea and made sure she would be okay to drive home.

Case #2: Mr. F was told he was having another heart attack, and he needed to be taken to the intensive care unit immediately. Mr. F's friend told the emergency room doctor that Mr. F did not want to be put on any machines. The emergency room doctor asked Mr. F if he wanted to die. Mr. F was too short of breath to answer. The doctor dismissed the friend's comment because he was not family and did not have durable power of attorney. Mr. F. was eventually able to communicate with the doctor and made his wishes clear that he did not want to be placed on any machines. The doctor reluctantly agreed to the requested DNR status and transferred the patient to a medical unit with telemetry.

On arrival to the floor, Mr. F's friend was told he needed to go home because visiting hours were over. Mr. F was connected to the telemetry monitor, placed on 2 L nasal cannula, and admitted. The nurse was frustrated that Mr. F could not answer the admission questions because he was so short of breath. She turned his oxygen up to 4 L and planned to finish the assessment when Mr. F was more rested. The nurse asked if there was anything else Mr. F needed. Mr. F told the nurse he was having chest pain and asked for pain medication.

The nurse reviewed Mr. F's orders and saw he was a DNR. She returned to Mr. F's room and medicated him for pain as ordered. She left the room and turned off the lights. Mr. F felt frightened and alone but did not want to bother the busy nurse. After 2 hours, the nurse noted that Mr. F's heart rhythm and breathing were becoming more irregular on the monitor. She went to Mr. F's room to check on him. He did not respond to her calling his name or to touch. Mr. F was grimacing, but the nurse ignored the change, thinking medicating Mr. F now would only cause him to die quicker. She left the room, and Mr. F was again alone. The nurse informed the other nurses on the unit that "Mr. F was on his way out."

The nurse decided to call family and notify them of Mr. F's pending death. There was no next of kin listed; only the friend they sent home earlier. The nurse called the friend and told him Mr. F might not make it through the night and he should come back to the hospital if he wanted to be with him. Mr. F died alone in the darkened room before his friend could arrive.

When Mr. F's friend arrived, he was told at the nurse's station that Mr. F had died. No one noticed the friend's grief as the staff hurried to complete their tasks to end their shift. The friend was given paperwork to sign and asked what funeral home needed to be called.

Case #3: Mr. F was told he was having another heart attack; but given his already weakened heart and kidneys, he was not a candidate for aggressive measures. Mr. F knew he was dying and asked to just be made comfortable. The emergency room doctor knew it was too late in the evening to call hospice, so he admitted Mr. F to a medical floor on comfort measures.

On arrival to the floor, Mr. F was placed on 2 L nasal cannula and a morphine PCA of 1 mg every hour with 0.5 mg boluses available every 15 minutes as needed. Mr. F's friend helped with the admission questions. The nurse provided extra blankets for the friend and told Mr. F she would be back to check on them.

Mr. F and his friend sat in silence and watched a hunting show on TV. The friend saw how Mr. F was struggling to breathe and asked if he should call the nurse. Mr. F told his friend not to bother the nurse because she was too busy. The friend sat and listened to Mr. F's suffering. When the nurse did return, Mr. F was unresponsive, and his friend was in tears. The nurse tried to console the friend and told him Mr. F did not have much longer to live. She asked if anyone else needed to be called. Mr. F shook his head slowly and said no. The nurse left the room and told the charge nurse that her patient was near death. The charge nurse told the nurse she needed to take another patient since Mr. F was dying and she had less work now.

The nurse became busy with her new admission and could not get back to check on Mr. F. A few hours later, Mr. F's friend came to the nurse's desk to tell them Mr. F was dead and that he was going home.

Case #4: The emergency room physician was certified in palliative medicine. He knew Mr. F was not a candidate for any aggressive procedures, and he did not have a living will. The physician pulled up a chair to discuss Mr. F's goals of care. He actively listened as Mr. F made his wishes clear. He nodded with empathy and understanding and suggested Mr. F spend the night in the inpatient hospice until arrangements could be made in the morning to send him home with hospice following, if that was what he desired. Mr. F agreed to the plan and stated he knew he was dying. He was placed on a morphine PCA at 1 mg/hr with as needed boluses of 0.5 mg every 15 minutes as needed and oxygen per nasal cannula at 2 L/min. Admission assessments were completed in the ER, and a report was called to the in-patient hospice unit so Mr. F could be taken directly to his room to rest.

The nurse working in the in-patient hospice unit pulled the CARES tool–based standing orders and utilized the CARES tool to plan her care.

Comfort: The nurse asked Mr. F if his chest pain had improved. He said no, and the nurse asked if it was getting worse. Mr. F nodded in agreement. The nurse instructed Mr. F on how to give himself a bolus with his PCA and about her plan to monitor the number of boluses he needed to be comfortable so the basal rate could be adjusted every 4 hours if needed. Mr. F felt better after the bolus and was comforted by the nurse's attention and kindness. The nurse made sure Mr. F was comfortable, then she asked if she could speak to his friend in the hall. Mr. F's friend followed the nurse out of the room to a comfortable lounge. He was offered something to drink, and the nurse sat down in a chair across from him. She kept direct eye contact and reached out to pat the friend's arm occasionally as she asked if he understood what was going on. The nurse confirmed there were no additional family members to call and invited the friend to stay with Mr. F as long as he liked. When the friend asked if the nurse thought Mr. F would die tonight, the nurse patted the friend's hand reassuringly and said, "Yes, it is very possible Mr. F could die tonight. I will be available to you and Mr. F to help you through this and to keep Mr. F comfortable."

Airway: The nurse noted Mr. F's breathing was becoming more labored. She obtained a fan and positioned it to gently blow across the side of Mr. F's face. She gave a dose of glycopyrrolate to help control his increasing oropharyngeal secretions and positioned him in a more comfortable sitting position. The nurse held his hand as she asked if his breathing had improved. Mr. F was too short of breath to speak at this point but was able to whisper, "Yes." The nurse told Mr. F she would stay with him and help him in any way she could. She told Mr. F she would not let him suffer. Mr. F nodded in appreciation and gently squeezed her hand.

Restlessness: Mr. F became very restless and was slow to answer the nurse to deny any increase in his pain. The nurse completed a quick physical assessment and noted that Mr. F's bladder was significantly distended. The nurse inserted a urinary catheter per the CARES order set and obtained 1,200 cc of cloudy concentrated urine. Mr. F's restlessness improved slightly, but the nurse observed the way he kept a tight grasp of his blanket and heard him call out at random for his now deceased wife. The nurse gave haloperidol IV, and Mr. F began to rest comfortably. She lowered the lights and reassured the friend. The nurse encouraged the friend to speak softly to Mr. F and tell him he was at his side. She explained how hearing was believed to be the last sense to deteriorate in the dying process and could be a calming effect. The friend pulled his chair closer, held Mr. F's hand and spoke softly about their last hunting trip and how he would always be here for his friend. The nurse stood by the friend and patted his shoulder softly. She explained the restlessness Mr. F was experiencing was normal and that he was not suffering.

Emotional support: The friend was visibly upset, and the nurse listened to his concerns and how deeply he was going to miss his friend. As the friend began to cry, the nurse sat in silence with him. She told him Mr. F was lucky to have such a special friend to keep him company. The friend smiled and wiped his tears with a tissue the nurse gave him. Mr. F continued to rest comfortably. He no longer spoke, and his breathing was becoming more irregular. The friend shared that Mr. F's favorite hunting show was about to start. The nurse suggested she turn on the TV to provide familiar sounds that could further comfort Mr. F. The friend agreed and began explaining what was happening on the show as he held Mr. F's hand. Mr. F was now having long episodes of apnea, but his face had softened to almost a smile as the friend continued to talk and laugh about something on the TV. The nurse checked on them frequently and made sure they were aware she was available. The nurse returned to find the friend had fallen asleep. She spoke gently to Mr. F and noted no response. His skin was now cool and mottled, and his blood pressure was barely audible at 42/palpation. The apnea episodes continued to extend, and Mr. F stopped breathing and died peacefully with his friend at his side. The nurse gently woke the friend and told him Mr. F had just died. She hugged the friend as he sobbed and told him how comforting it must have been to have a best friend at his side. The friend sat holding Mr. F's hand and the nurse sat quietly next to him. The friend spoke after a few moments. He thanked the nurse and said he needed to make some calls. The nurse asked if anyone else would be coming in to see Mr. F. The friend shook his head no and said he would call the funeral home. The nurse asked if he needed help with the phone calls and the friend whispered "no" and walked out of the room.

Self-care: The nurse was touched by Mr. F's peacefulness and the close relationship he had with his friend. She became tearful as she shared the events that transpired around the hunting show. The other nurses on the unit gave her hugs and asked if she would be okay to drive home. The nurse said she would but decided first to get a cup of coffee. The nurse had a self-care ritual to sit outside, relax with a cup of coffee, and review her day. She was honored to help Mr. F on his final journey and took pride in knowing she made his last few hours comfortable. The nurse absorbed the beautiful morning and said a short prayer for Mr. F and his friend.

Case #5: Mr. F's cardiac enzymes were elevated, and he was told he was having a heart attack and needed to be taken to the intensive care unit immediately. Mr. F's friend told the emergency room doctor that Mr. F did not want to be put on any machines. The emergency room doctor asked Mr. F if he wanted to die. Mr. F was too short of breath to answer. The doctor dismissed the friend's comment since he was not family and did not have durable power of attorney. Mr. F's breathing continued to decline, and the emergency room physician intubated him and placed him on a ventilator. Mr. F became increasingly restless and tried to pull out the breathing tube. He was restrained and sedated. The friend became increasingly upset and told the doctor again, "This is not what he wanted." The emergency room doctor stated, "If this isn't what he wanted, then why did he come to the emergency room? The breathing machine is just temporary until we can stabilize him, then we will remove it."

The friend shook his head in disbelief and sat down next to Mr. F. The friend followed Mr. F to the intensive care unit when three nurses transported him by gurney, pushing monitors and IV pumps, and bagging Mr. F because the sedation he was given prevented him from breathing on his own.

The friend watched in disbelief as Mr. F's room became crowded with medical staff rushing to draw blood, connect IV tubing to pumps, and hook up monitoring equipment. Mr. F was almost unrecognizable under all the equipment. The friend was told he needed to go to the waiting room. They were taking Mr. F to the cath lab and would notify him when he returned.

The cardiologist wanted to place a heart-assist device called an intra-aortic balloon pump (IABP) to allow Mr. F's heart to rest and heal. It was intended to support him through his heart attack. Mr. F woke and tried to get the doctor's attention to ask him to stop, but he was again sedated. The IABP connection catheter was inserted through Mr. F's artery in his right groin. The device was working well, and Mr. F's heart stabilized. A staff nurse in the cath lab noticed Mr. F's right leg turning blue and cold. The cardiologist knew this meant the IABP catheter was blocking blood flow down Mr. F's leg. He made the choice to monitor the leg closely to buy time to get Mr. F through the most critical time of his heart attack. Orders were given to keep Mr. F heavily sedated so he couldn't move his leg for the next 24 hours.

The friend sat next to Mr. F and sadly shook his head. He asked the nurse if he could put Mr. F's favorite hunting show on the TV. The nurse felt it was a bad idea because it might be too stimulating. Right now Mr. F needed to be perfectly still, and she suggested the friend go home since visiting hours were almost over. She promised to call the friend if there were any changes in Mr. F's condition. The friend got up and gave Mr. F's hand a squeeze and told him he would see him in the morning.

Mr. F's leg grew more and more mottled until a decision was made to take him to the operating room and remove the IABP catheter and try to repair any damage to his artery. Once Mr. F was positioned on the surgical table, the device was removed, and his heart became too weak to beat normally. He went into cardiac arrest and the operating team worked to resuscitate him for more than 2 hours before the cardiologist pronounced him dead. Mr. F was taken directly to the morgue because his bed in intensive care was needed for another admission.

The friend arrived early the next morning hoping Mr. F had a restful night. The friend walked into the room and stared at the stranger in Mr. F's bed. When the friend asked where Mr. F was, the nurse on duty said she had no idea. The friend became angry and the nurse called security to escort him out of the building.

CASE STUDY SUMMARY

The presentation of the five scenarios was intended to demonstrate the impact good communication skills, an understanding of basic palliative care and end-of-life training, and establishing individualized goals of care can have on patient outcomes. The scenarios also demonstrate how the CARES tool can be used to prompt the nurse, and to help anticipate the commonly needed orders to more effectively support the dying and their families.

An emphasis must be placed on the establishment of patient-driven goals of care. This can only be achieved through communication and compassionate listening. Care should be based on the needs of the individual and not on the health care provider's schedule.

The term "family" is used throughout this text. It encompasses friends, loved ones, and anyone who plays a significant role in the life of the dying individual. They are often in a position to provide valuable insight into the needs and wishes of the dying, and the health care provider should consider this information when attempting to act in the best interest of the dying.

The scenarios provide stark contrasts on the use of compassion, empathy, and the ability and willingness to demonstrate basic acts of kindness and humanity. It becomes the decision of health care providers to act as advocates and to decide how they want to interact with their patients and families. It is my hope that these choices will always be guided by compassion.

A PERSONAL SHARING

I want to emphasize that, no matter how earnest the effort, some patients will not experience a peaceful death and the importance of self-care for the health care provider. The following is an example of the gifts and challenges nurses can obtain when they open their heart to a dying individual and his or her family. This is a story about Mike and how he provided an opportunity for me to grow spiritually and to renew my resolve that no one should ever have to die in pain.

Mike was a 46-year-old kind and loving father of twin boys who were about to graduate from high school. He was happily married and had loving parents all wanting to be actively involved with his care. Mike had metastatic renal cancer to his spine. I was treating him for chronic pain in his back and right groin. Eventually, a decision was made to implant an intrathecal access pain pump to better manage Mike's pain. This was successful and for 1 month Mike's pain was controlled.

Mike began having more difficulty walking and was developing increasing edema of both legs. I would agree to reprogram Mike's pain pump, because any activity was becoming increasingly painful for this sweet and gentle man.

Eventually, Mike's pain became so severe in his right groin that he would scream in pain. After several ineffective pump solution changes and reprogramming, he was hospitalized. A diagnosis of lepto-meningeal metastasis was confirmed and a spinal cord stimulator was implanted in addition to the intrathecal pain pump. The combination therapy provided Mike with 2 weeks of controlled pain relief and then this treatment, too, began to fail.

No amount of IV opioids could control Mike's pain as he began to scream to be allowed to die. He was admitted to a hospital closer to his home as his pain became so severe he could not tolerate the 1-hour drive to my facility. I was told by the wife that palliative care was following and they promised to do their best to make Mike comfortable.

I called the wife on the following Monday, only to find Mike was discharged home on hospice as the palliative care doctor became uncomfortable with the large amount of opioids Mike required and that his pain was still not under control.

Mike was taken home and never stopped screaming. His children were devastated and his wife was furious that no one could control her husband's pain. Hospice came to the home and through the night gave Mike bolus after bolus of opioids without effect until his breathing began to decline. Mike was continuing to scream when he could catch his breath and died just moments before I called.

Mike was a classic candidate for palliative sedation and should have been placed on benzodiazepines along with the opioids. His pain would still be present but his brain would not have processed the stimulus as pain. Mike would have become unresponsive sooner, but he would not have screamed in pain with his last breath. My regret is that I was not there to help him.

It is this regret, this sense of failure I wanted to share and to emphasize the need for self-care. Yes, I will always be frustrated by the painful death Mike and his family were forced to endure. In Chapter 11 the need to review this type of painful event is emphasized.

I realized the pedestal Mike and his family placed me on was of their own belief and not based on reality. I am not all-knowing and I probably would not have provided anything different. Palliative sedation is ethically challenging, but because of Mike I now know that I will not hesitate providing it in the future.

I also realized I was limited by the family's choice to go to a closer hospital. I needed to accept I did the best I could, and I struggled to find some meaning from this experience. After much anger, frustration, tears, and sharing with coworkers, I arrived at the realization that the positive takeaway was the journey.

For just over 6 months I was blessed to know this courageous, funny, beautiful man and his wonderful family. I provided comfort and helped give Mike some quality for the time he had remaining. I cared about Mike as a human being and reinforced his sense of dignity and self-worth. I was honored that I got to know him and humbled at his willingness to be vulnerable and frightened with me. Our last interaction occurred just 2 weeks earlier when I filled his pain pump. Mike was sitting in his wheelchair grimacing in pain. He leaned toward me and placed his head on my shoulder and cried. I hugged this sweet man and told him "I wished I could be of more help, and that I would always try to be there for him."

I think that last statement is what haunts me. I needed to let go of my sense of failure as I could not be everywhere, especially when he was admitted to another hospital and cared for by a hospice out of my area. I needed to identify how realistic I was being, and I recognized my sense of failure was not based on reality.

I am a better nurse practitioner and a better human being for having known Mike. That is the positive from this and any relationship I have been lucky enough to establish with the dying. Good self-care is needed to embrace the gifts obtained from these experiences. I encourage caregivers not to avoid this opportunity. There is a need to submit to your grief and to allow yourself to be human. I do not want to avoid the opportunity to get close to my patients, so I must accept that grief will accompany my choice. I embrace the fact that when my heart is broken, it is open to take in painful and at the same time beautiful experiences such as the one I was honored to receive from Mike and his family. I am somehow stronger and a better person because of the journey we took together.

I share this experience to honor Mike, to help me work through my grief and find meaning, and to share the challenges and the gifts that can be obtained when caring for the dying. I encourage nurses to find a way to open their hearts and to grow when given similar opportunities.

PART IV

Barriers and Challenges

CHAPTER 17

Changing a Culture

The CARES tool can only be effective if utilized. This remains a challenge because many health care institutions still embrace the belief that death is a mark of failure, or a dreaded event to be ignored, and therefore it is never openly discussed. Consider how a body is transported off a hospital unit. A cart with a special cover is used, doors are closed so as not to upset others on the unit, family members are asked to remain in their rooms, and a back-hall route is utilized to transport the body to the morgue as unobtrusively as possible. The hope is for no one to notice and for no one to be confronted by death. Our culture does not consider death a normal part of life. Imagine my surprise when I was told about a veteran's hospital that announced the death of an individual over the hospital's address system and all available staff and all able persons being cared for at the facility were asked to line the halls as the body was removed and taken out through the front entrance to a waiting funeral home transport vehicle. The individuals able to attend not only came in large numbers, but saluted as the body was rolled past them. Imagine, the body was taken out the front door in plain sight of everyone! This is a very unusual policy and one I do not see many hospitals imitating in the near future, but it does emphasize how secretive and close-minded our culture is about death.

Two major steps are necessary to change our health care culture's denial of death and embrace the decision to provide quality evidence-based care for the dying and their families. First, it will require the acceptance and willingness to consult a palliative care team to assist in providing evidence-based symptom management for the terminally ill. Second, it will require the education, embracement, and advocacy of nursing for it to be successful.

THE IMPORTANCE OF THE PALLIATIVE CARE
MULTIDISCIPLINARY TEAM

When the need for a palliative care consult is discussed, many medical professionals and society in general automatically associate the decision with a premature sense of giving up and a loss of hope (Ferrell & Coyle, 2010). There is often a direct association with hospice, end of life (EOL), and dying. This overwhelming emotional, cultural, and psychological association greatly diminishes the likelihood of a palliative care consult and greatly reduces the quality of care that can be provided to a terminally ill person and his or her family.

The ideal situation for the terminally ill would be to consult the palliative care multidisciplinary team to assist with symptom management as early in their treatment as possible. The aim would be to establish personalized goals of care, and support an improved quality of life for individuals as they define it, and for as long as they require. There is no average time frame; a terminally ill individual can still have a life expectancy of many years. The involvement of a palliative care team does not imply the patient will die soon. Unfortunately, it is common to consult the palliative care team when an individual has only days or hours to live. I truly believe this is where the negative association comes in. Palliative care is much more effective if started early. Getting a palliative care team involved early to provide supportive care and evidence-based symptom management actually allows a focus on quality of life. In fact, research has now shown individuals actually live longer when they receive palliative care (Swetz & Kamal, 2012). Palliative care medicine addresses the entire scope of treatment and support required for the care of a chronic illness, from diagnosis to death. EOL care is a service provided by palliative care, but it is only one of several supportive measures they can provide.

The palliative care team would eventually focus on comfort care as the patient transitions to the actively dying phase of his or her disease. With the help of a skilled and supportive palliative care interdisciplinary team, a seamless transition into care of the actively dying can occur.

Palliative care, and in particular EOL care, is a natural fit for nurses. Nurses could extend the reach of palliative care to all patients as the basic tenets of palliative care are "integral to the scope and standards of professional nursing and all specialty areas of nursing practice" (McHugh, Arnold, & Buschman, 2012, p. 140). For a change to occur in the standards of care for the hospitalized dying, nurses must become advocates for the individuals and their families under their care. Nurses must become skilled providers in palliative care and more specifically, EOL care.

A slow change in culture is occurring throughout the country as hospitals incorporate the concepts of palliative care medicine into their standards of care to meet increasing patient care demands of the chronically ill.

Facilitating a change in a hospital's culture and service delivery requires the utilization and implementation of organizational change theory and incorporation of adult learning principles (Boshoff, 2005; Knowles et al., 2005). Factors influencing culture change must be embraced and the development of new service strategies will be required to maintain financial sustainability for many health care institutions. For a change in culture to be successfully integrated into an existing organization, it must also be viewed as nonthreatening and respectful of an institution's existing culture (Rogers, 2003).

Several theories of change can assist in the cultural change process for an organization to incorporate palliative and EOL care into their standards of practice. Boshoff (2005) identified organizational change as a complex and challenging process of ongoing responses to continuous changes that occur in our environment. Price (2008) noted that understanding the change experience and retaining a sense of self-worth and professional skills can greatly assist health care workers as they adapt to change. Kurt Lewin's (Burnes, 2004) three-step Change model, Elisabeth Kübler-Ross's (1969) Five Stages of Grief, and William Bridges's (2004) Managing Transitions theory provide a general overview of a successful change process. John Kotter's (2012) Eight-Step Change theory and Everett Rogers's (2003) Diffusion of Innovation supply a detailed framework on how to bring about a successful change in culture (Robinson Hickman, 2010; Rogers, 2003).

KURT LEWIN AND ELISABETH KÜBLER-ROSS

The first step of Kurt Lewin's three-step process involves unfreezing. This phase is representative of most change theories as the need for change must be identified and a readiness or willingness for change must be established. Nurses are verbalizing a desire to learn how to more effectively manage the needs of the dying and their families. Lewin believed the status quo or the individual's equilibrium must be disrupted (unfrozen) before old behavior can be unlearned and new behavior adopted (Burnes, 2004). This is a very difficult phase because it requires letting go of comfortable routines and embracing new techniques. Nurses are no longer willing to feel abandoned and unsupported by management and physicians when caring for a dying patient. It is no longer ethically acceptable to ignore the needs of a dying patient. Nurses feel justified acting as advocates and, as Lewin observed as a requirement for unfreezing, they feel "safe from loss and humiliation before they can accept the new information and reject old behaviors" (p. 985).

William Bridges's (2004) Managing Transitions theory included the recognition of "endings," where there is a sense of no longer being able to turn back, and a realization that things will no longer be the same. There is resistance and a desire to hold on to the status quo. Bridges (2004) described this phase as "passage ritual," dependent upon social reality and a natural ending process that requires disengagement, dismantling, disidentification, disenchantment, and disorientation.

Dr. Kübler-Ross's Five Stages of Grief can be applied to this initiation of a change process because a form of grief exists when a culture is forced to change or adapt. The process requires a letting go of comfortable and deeply ingrained methods of patient care. There is "anger" and "bargaining" as the health care staff struggle to embrace palliative care and incorporate it into everyday practice (Kübler-Ross, 1969).

Bridges (2004) emphasized that endings are like dying experiences and strongly agreed with Dr. Kübler-Ross. He believed endings challenge our basic sense of who we are, the familiar, and the known. Time must be allowed to experience an ending for a letting-go process to occur and a transition to the next phase of change.

Organizational change can assist in this ending/unfreezing/grieving process for health care staff through educational opportunities that allow for the acquisition and internalization of information (Boshoff, 2005). Staff can learn improved care methods for symptom management of the terminally ill and dying and accept the need to incorporate the new behaviors and skills into their daily practice. Not all health care providers will make this transition as quickly as others, so ongoing education and role modeling will be essential.

Once there is an acceptance that palliative care can improve care for the chronically ill, dying, as a new phase of change, begins. This phase is identified by Kurt Lewin as the "moving phase" because endings, unfreezing, and grieving processes create the motivation for change but do not supply a strategy to achieve the change goal. New strategies must be implemented to drive the desired change (Burnes, 2004). All options to ensure successful integration of palliative care principles need to be explored to promote learning and acceptance as health care providers continue to struggle to let go of past behaviors and beliefs. This could be the point when prior staffing plans can no longer be supported if a nurse caring for a dying individual and his or her family continues to receive an additional assignment based on the antiquated belief that there is nothing to be done for a dying patient.

The moving phase is supported by Kübler-Ross's (1969) phases of bargaining and depression as health care providers continue to struggle to adjust to the changes in practice and grieve over the loss of the familiar. Change can be painful, it is a common human response to hold on to the familiar rather than take on a new method of resolving a situation. William Bridges (2004) describes this time as being in the "neutral zone." It is a time of uncertainty, like being in a fog, or an adjustment phase when new skills are learned but are not fully embraced. Boshoff (2005) notes change requires a problem-solving process that:

1. Identifies a problem or recognizes a need for change
2. Provides a thorough investigation of the problem
3. Recommends evidence-based strategies to solve the problem
4. Utilizes principles of adult learning and active involvement of all participants
5. Requires critical reflection and evaluation of strategy effectiveness
6. Implements any needed changes or adjustments identified from the evaluation process

Ownership for change must occur for all participants. Boshoff (2005) noted, "People tend to support what they have helped to create" (p. 150). A successful palliative care program that has a foundation in nurse advocacy will require commitment and a shared vision from all key stakeholders.

Organizational change must start with education and the implementation of adult learning principles (Boshoff, 2005; Knowles et al., 2005). Health care staff cannot and will not embrace a change in patient care delivery without education, encouragement, and the personal belief that a change is necessary (Knowles et al., 2005). The findings of Barrere, Durkin, and LaCoursiere (2008) echoed some of the four major tenets of Carl Rogers's student-centered approach to education.

1. An individual cannot be taught directly; learning must be facilitated
2. An individual only learns what is perceived as personally important
3. Learning requires the assimilation of knowledge and a resultant change in behavior
4. Individuals are resistant to change

The final phase of Kurt Lewin's three-step theory of change is refreezing. This occurs when the new change is accepted and becomes part of the culture. Burnes (2004) described this step in Lewin's theory as an attempt to "stabilize the group at a new quasi-stationary equilibrium in order to ensure that the new behaviors are relatively safe from regression" (p. 986). Lewin believed a new behavior must be congruent with current cultural norms, behaviors, and supported by the existing environment of the learner to be successful (Burnes, 2004). Lewin's refreezing phase closely resembles and supports the major tenets just discussed in Carl Rogers's student-centered approach to education and adult learning.

Lewin's refreezing step is further defined by Kübler-Ross's (1969) stage of acceptance as part of the Five Stages of Grief theory. Health care providers can now accept that previous methods of caring for the chronically and terminally ill are insufficient and begin to embrace palliative care medicine as their new standard of practice. This is a continued period of readjustment and learning that allows for personal and professional growth.

William Bridges describes this phase as a "new beginning," the establishment of "hope," and the embracing of a "new reality" (Bridges, 2004; Robinson Hickman, 2010). Price (2008) noted understanding the change experience and retaining a sense of self-worth and professional skills can greatly assist health care workers as they adapt to change. Unfortunately, health care typically changes because of "revolution rather than evolution" (Price, 2008, p. 51). The greatest driving force to change a culture and adapt palliative care into standard medical practice is our aging society, our increasing population of the chronically ill, and the necessity to provide quality evidence-based care to an ever-increasing well-informed patient population.

Education and advanced planning to embrace a palliative care program can minimize disruption, feelings of losing control, and reduce the negative impact on self-esteem that can occur with abrupt mandated health care changes (Price, 2008). When change occurs gradually, the need for coping assistance and counseling is diminished. This education tactic addresses two more tenets of Carl Rogers's student-centered approach to education: the learning requirements of a relaxed nonthreatening environment and a reduction of the learner's fears to promote understanding of concepts and the learning process (Knowles et al., 2005; Price, 2008). A gradual change in a health care delivery system through education, encouragement, and the establishment of a shared vision will allow health care providers to feel in control and to champion the need and the desire to provide quality palliative care (Barrere et al., 2008; Knowles et al., 2005; Price, 2008).

EVERETT M. ROGERS AND JOHN KOTTER

A more detailed plan for implementing a change in culture to embrace palliative care medicine can be obtained through the use of Everett M. Rogers's (2003) conceptual model Diffusion of Innovation and John Kotter's (2012) Eight-Step Change model. They both provide a very in-depth theoretical framework for change that echoes many of the recommendations previously discussed by Lewin, Kübler-Ross, Price, Boshoff, and Bridges.

Rogers (2003) defined innovation as a desired change, improvement, or object that is perceived as new. This newness can be expressed as knowledge, persuasion, or a decision to adopt an alternate method or approach. Both Rogers (2003) and Kotter (2012) envisioned change as an ongoing process that requires many important elements or components to be successful.

Rogers's (2003) Diffusion of Innovation theory has five essential concepts and six required components that must be compatible with the needs and requirements of the current culture for diffusion of an innovation to occur. Kotter's (2012) Change model identifies eight tasks that must be completed for organizational change to occur and be sustained.

The desired change to integrate palliative care medicine into an existing hospital culture can be accomplished through the use of Rogers's (2003) initial five concepts of advantage, compatibility, complexity, trialability, and observability. The six necessary components to ensure a successful change according to Rogers are the availability of needed resources, the establishment of communication channels, time availability, compatibility with existing social systems, the capture of a critical mass, and the establishment of champions. All of Rogers's concepts and necessary components for his Diffusion of Innovation theory are supported and further enhanced by Kotter's (2012) eight requirements for successful change, which are: establishing a sense of urgency, creating a guiding coalition, developing a vision and strategy, communicating the change vision, empowering broad-based action, generating short-term wins, consolidating gains and producing more change, and anchoring new approaches in the culture. The integration of the two change theories can be applied to changing the care delivery for chronically ill and dying patients in a hospital setting with the introduction of palliative care medicine as a standard practice could occur as follows.

Advantage: Rogers (2003) defined an advantage as a benefit, gain, or improvement the innovation or change project will provide. Kotter (2012) would emphasize the acknowledgment of an advantage by attaching a sense of urgency. The change must be viewed as important, necessary, and urgently needed to obtain the energy and willingness of stakeholders to support. The advantage of implementing a palliative care program would demonstrate the progressive focus of the hospital and their willingness to incorporate current research to improve hospital care. Palliative care has become a fundamental component of medicine as it addresses patients and their families holistically with a focus on quality of life and the alleviation of adverse symptoms (City of Hope & AACN, 2012). It is synonymous with nursing because the primary focus of palliative care is to provide culturally meaningful compassionate care, which incorporates strong communication skills and patient advocacy (McHugh et al., 2012). Nursing could take the lead in this change process by becoming a strong patient advocate, improving communication, and re-establishing the importance of spirituality and holistic patient care. The urgency could be based on the ever-increasing numbers of chronically ill patients and the inadequate care they are currently receiving. The desire to prevent unnecessary suffering should be emphasized and the desire to no longer accept providing suboptimal care.

Compatibility: Rogers (2003) notes that compatibility is achieved when a change project is well suited, like minded, or well matched to the current needs and social focus of an institution, culture, or group. Kotter (2012) would support this need for compatibility by emphasizing a shared vision to provide the highest quality of care possible for patients. The hospital has a long-term established curative culture and education will be essential to promote an understanding of the difference between palliative medicine and hospice for health care professionals (Swetz & Kamal, 2012). Health care providers need to understand that palliative care medicine is designed to complement the physician's efforts to treat their patients through symptom management and holistic-focused support during the chronic disease process. A health care provider trained in palliative care medicine can address the often time-consuming unmet symptom management needs of patients and their families. They can ensure time will be provided to actually listen to the patient, answer any questions, and provide holistic support to address fears and concerns. They can reduce the strain on the primary physician's time and allow them to remain focused on the disease treatment plan (Bruera & Hui, 2012).

Complexity: Rogers (2003) addresses the complexity of a change project, and focuses on the need to reduce perceived difficulties or intricacies of implementation and obtaining necessary resources. The complexity of a project could be further reduced by Kotter's (2012) recommendation to provide support and involvement by a guiding coalition to champion the change and reduce any barriers. Providing palliative care training is not complex. Palliative care could be nurse driven and education of symptom management and holistic patient and family care practices could be established through mandatory education (McHugh et al., 2012). Nurses would become skilled in communication and patient advocacy. They would be trained to request patient-specific comfort orders, supply extended patient education, and provide psychosocial support to their patients and families (Ferrell & Coyle, 2010). Any advanced or complicated palliative care medicine issues could be referred to a dedicated palliative care team available for consultation (Bruera & Hui, 2012). The palliative care team would be composed of experienced pain and symptom management specialists, social workers, dieticians, spiritual counselors, psychiatrists, psychologists, and child-life specialists (Bruera & Hui, 2012). Social workers would act as overall patient advocates and encourage palliative care team consults as identified. The greatest challenges would be to provide and reinforce nursing education in palliative care, educating all medical staff on palliative care medicine, and motivating physicians to utilize the palliative care team for more complex symptom management (Bruera & Hui, 2012). All necessary resources should be available to the medical center, and all needed educational resources and training opportunities should be obtainable within the institution.

Trialability: Rogers (2003) refers to the trialability of a change project as the anticipated challenges of organizing a study or assessment of the possible effectiveness of the proposed change project. It is the degree a change concept can undergo experimentation and be tested over time (Rogers, 2003). Kotter (2012) echoes the need to seek the acceptance of initiating a research-based palliative care training program through communicating the vision to all stakeholders and obtaining their much-needed understanding and support. Hospital administration, acting as part of the supportive coalition discussed earlier, would be required to act as the driving force to mandate education and training of all health care staff.

Observability: Rogers (2003) defines observability as the level of perceived difference or modification to current practice to be anticipated. It is the "degree to which the results of an innovation are visible to others" (Rogers, 2003, p. 258). Kotter (2012) again concurs with Rogers and addresses observability through the recommendation of empowering change champions to confront and resolve any barriers to providing palliative care medicine hospital-wide. The use of a dedicated coalition can supply or assist in the development of super-users or change champions that can effectively role model how to provide palliative care. Their presence should be integrated into all health care groups to motivate and sustain the desired change in practice through example. Observability can be further ensured as nursing administrations adopt a patient care philosophy based on palliative care medicine as part of their plan to pursue Magnet Status and hospital-wide palliative care certification. Nursing administration would need to fully embrace palliative care medicine and identify its tenets as the core of their patient care philosophy. Yearly skills validation will need to include palliative care skills such as patient advocacy, communication, and symptom management. Ongoing research should be done to equate the adoption of palliative care principles and increased patient and health care staff satisfaction. The effectiveness of a change in culture must be readily observable and viewed as essential to improving care of the chronically ill by the health care staff for a change in culture to occur (Kotter, 2012; Rogers, 2003).

Once the five concepts of Diffusion of Innovation are satisfied, Rogers (2003) recommended six necessary components to insure a successful change as previously discussed. The components of Rogers's theory are again supported and made more complete by Kotter's (2012) eight-step approach. A table was developed to show how Kotter's theory can complement Rogers's six necessary components of the availability of needed resources, the establishment of communication channels, time availability, compatibility with existing social systems, the capturing of a critical mass, and the establishment of champions (see Table 17.1).

TABLE 17.1
Comparison of Rogers's Essential Components
and Kotter's Change Process

ROGERS'S SIX NECESSARY COMPONENTS	SIX OF KOTTER'S EIGHT STEPS FOR TRANSFORMATION
Necessary resources	Establishing a sense of urgency
	Creating a guiding coalition
	Empowering broad-based action
Communication channels	Communicating the change vision
	Developing a vision and strategy
	Creating a guiding coalition
Time availability	Creating a guiding coalition
	Developing a vision and strategy
	Empowering broad-based action
Compatibility with social systems	Creating a guiding coalition
	Developing a vision and strategy
	Communicating the change vision
	Empowering broad-based action
Capturing a critical mass	Establishing a sense of urgency
	Creating a guiding coalition
	Developing a vision and strategy
	Communicating the change vision
	Empowering broad-based action
	Generating short-term wins
Establishment of champions	Creating a guiding coalition
	Communicating the change vision
	Empowering broad-based action

Rogers (2003) advocates for the availability of needed resources to be confirmed for a change in practice to successfully occur. No project is possible without the supplies, equipment, and personnel to achieve the desired outcome. The members of Kotter's (2012) guiding coalition have a similar role as Rogers's champions. Members must be strong advocates for making palliative care medicine a standard of care by ensuring all necessary materials required to provide education and training in palliative care are available and continue to act as role models to promote acceptance of the planned improvement in care. The guiding coalition can reinforce the sense of urgency as a method to obtain any necessary resources and empower nurses to champion the change. The additional support will help to remove any obstacles to the education process so essential for this change. Rogers (2003) cites the establishment of communication channels as essential to the success and continued daily practice of a proposed change. Kotter (2012) also references the importance of communicating. He focused on the need for communicating a clear vision that would require the development of a vision strategy, and persons specifically trained to provide information. These individuals could be obtained through the guiding coalition or change champions. The incorporation of palliative care medicine as a standard of practice will require clear and open communication to prevent misunderstandings, misdirection, and promote use of individual skills and expertise to achieve desired goals (Rogers, 2003). All parties must embrace the change vision and understand the goals and direction of the change project. This can only be achieved through strong communication channels.

Rogers (2003) viewed time availability as essential. He believed it must be obtained for any change project to be successful. Kotter's (2012) guiding coalition could positively influence health care providers as they become empowered through the sharing of the change vision, encouraged by example, and assisted with flexible scheduling options to attend the necessary education. If the issue is perceived as important, time will be made available. Weekend classes, videotaped classes, and classes posted on YouTube are all possibilities.

Rogers (2003) believed compatibility with existing social systems was essential and requires close examination of how palliative care medicine honors current institution priorities and social norms. Kotter (2012) supports this necessary component of change again through the establishment of a guiding coalition. Coalition members would have firsthand knowledge of cultural norms, informal leaders to acknowledge and seek support, and any other necessary culturally established issues requiring attention to achieve a lasting change in patient care.

The capturing of a critical mass is another essential component of change. The concept is embraced by both Rogers (2003) and Kotter (2012) as indispensable to the achievement of self-sustaining change. It requires a group of individuals who are supportive and active in the implementation of a change process to attain a size and social strength that results in the continued use or adoption of a desired change without further encouragement or persuasion (Rogers, 2003). Kotter (2012) recommends to not only achieve a critical mass but also celebrate it by acknowledging small gains within the group. A change may require 3 to 10 years to become a standard part of a culture. This often long course needs nurturing and the avoidance of complacency to be successful. Maintaining the energy required for the change process to continue will require the successful achievement of Kotter's (2012) sixth stage: the generation of short-term wins. Kotter believed that success no matter how insignificant should be recognized.

Kotter's (2012) remaining two stages, consolidating gains and producing more change and anchoring new approaches in the culture, continue to build on the successful change process. They provide a plan to sustain the desired change. This focus was not fully addressed by Rogers's (2003) Diffusion of Innovation theory. Kotter (2012) felt change is very fragile and caution should be used when celebrating a perceived successful change. The first evidence of performance improvement does not mean the desired change in practice will be sustained. A true change must "sink down deeply into a culture. An entire company could take three to ten years, new approaches are fragile and subject to regression" (p. 227). Evidence of accomplishing original goals and the presence of behavioral changes in health care staff must be verified. Often, a desired change is not sustained over time because the momentum was diminished by a false sense of victory, the urgency was not valued, the coalition lacked the necessary power, or the vision was unclear. Ongoing education for health care staff provided on a regular basis, the establishment of focus groups to discuss any difficulties or concerns, practice and ongoing training of new skills, recognizing the palliative care achievements of staff, and rewarding the desired behaviors can help to sustain the change in practice.

Nurses want to provide quality evidence-based palliative care. They are aware that their patients are suffering. Education is the key as "all nurses should have generalist palliative care knowledge and skills to provide guidance to patients and families regarding disease states, trajectories of illness, psychosocial support, discussion regarding advance directives, and symptom management" (McHugh et al., 2012, p. 143). Nurses throughout the country are already experiencing a sense of urgency.

Anchoring new approaches in the culture is the final step in Kotter's (2003) change plan. He emphasizes the importance of facilities continuing to explore new methods to improve practices and make the desired change a permanent part of the culture. Once a change process has become a part of the culture, it should be sustainable over time. Kotter (2003) noted that two important factors are required to anchor a change process within a culture:

1. Making a conscious effort to acknowledge specific behaviors and attitudes that demonstrate the benefits of the desired change over previous methods

2. Taking the time to ensure future management continues to support the desired change

Kotter (2003) wanted to emphasize sustaining a change in culture requires continuous nurturing and support. Failure to achieve any of the eight steps of change in Kotter's (2003) Transitional Change theory can result in resistance, frustration, and a failure to change. A false sense of accomplishment can be detrimental. Kotter compared it to "stumbling into a sink hole in the road to meaningful change. And, for a variety of reasons, even smart people don't just stumble into that hole. Sometimes, they jump in with both feet" (p. 236).

Promoting a change in the care and delivery provided to the chronically and terminally ill in a hospital setting is long overdue. Our aging society is demanding compassionate holistic care on the level of what hospice provides. It is a daunting task to change a predominately curative culture to one that embraces palliative care medicine and believes in its responsibility to provide a peaceful death.

The change theorists Lewin, Kübler-Ross, Bridges, Rogers, and Kotter provided recommendations for the plan to make palliative care medicine a standard of care in a hospital setting. Nurses are key to the success of this change project, as they must take on the role of patient advocate and change champion.

Change was identified as fragile, frightening, and often necessary for an improved quality of life. Time must be allowed to grieve over the loss of past methods of care and to embrace the urgency of implementing new technology while preserving the dignity, culture, and sense of control so necessary to the adult learner. The time has come for hospital settings to begin the process to fully embrace palliative care medicine into their daily practice, encourage nurses to act as advocates for the needs of the individuals under their care, and to support evidence-based care of the dying.

REFERENCES

Barrere, C. C., Durkin, A., & LaCoursiere, S. (2008). The influence of end-of-life education on nursing students. *International Journal of Nursing Education Scholarship, 5*(1), 1–18. Retrieved from CINAHL database.

Boshoff, K. (2005). Towards facilitating change in service delivery: An illustrative example. *Australian Occupational Therapy Journal, 52*(2), 149–159. Retrieved from CINAHL database.

Bridges, W. (2004). *Transitions: Making sense of life's changes.* (2nd ed.). Cambridge, MA: Perseus Book Group.

Bruera, E., & Hui, D. (2012). Conceptual models for integrating palliative care at cancer centers. *Journal of Palliative Medicine, 15*(11), 1261–1269. doi: 10.1089/jpm.2012.0174

Burnes, B. (2004). Kurt Lewin and the planned approach to change: A re-appraisal. *Journal of Management Studies, 41*(6), 977–1002.

City of Hope & AACN. (2012). *Final hours of life.* Module 8, End-of-Life Nursing Education Consortium (ELNEC). Washington, DC: AACN.

Knowles, M. S., Holton, E. F., & Swanson, R. A. (2005). *The adult learner: The definitive classic in adult education and human resource development* (6th ed.). San Diego, CA: Elsevier.

Kotter, P. J. (2012). *Leading change*. Boston, MA: Harvard Business Review Press.

Kübler-Ross, E. (1969). *On death & dying*. New York, NY: Simon and Schuster.

McHugh, M. E., Arnold, J., & Buschman, P. R. (2012). Nurses leading the response to the crisis of palliative care for vulnerable populations. *Nursing Economics, 30*(3), 140–147.

Price, B. (2008). Strategies to help nurses cope with change in the healthcare setting. *Nursing Standard, 22*(48), 50–56.

Robinson Hickman, G. (Ed.). (2010). *Leading organizations: Perspectives for a new era*. Los Angeles, CA: Sage.

Rogers, E. M. (2003). *Diffusion of innovations* (5th ed.). New York, NY: Free Press.

Swetz, K. M., & Kamal, A. H. (2012). In the clinic: Palliative care. *Annals of Internal Medicine, 2(16)*, 1–16.

CHAPTER 18

Translating Current Literature Into Evidence-Based Practice: The Role of the DNP

Embracing the role of a nurse practitioner with a doctorate in nursing practice (DNP) requires taking on the additional challenge of acting as an effective change agent. A DNP's primary role is to act as a bridge between research and the bedside nurse. Their educational focus is to become clinical experts and possess the ability to translate nursing research findings to clinical practice. The American Association of Colleges of Nursing (AACN) first endorsed the DNP program in 2004 in an effort to develop a clinically focused nursing doctorate program that recognized expert practitioners (Boland, Treston, & O'Sullivan, 2010). The DNP degree is now 10 years old and continues to establish its own uniqueness and importance as a respected terminal degree in nursing.

The DNP prepared nurse is typically a nurse practitioner, but an advanced practice master's prepared nurse can also become a DNP if he or she desires. Obtaining a DNP requires extensive clinical hours and a solid foundation in research interpretation. The ability to function as an expert in a clinical setting makes the DNP a valuable staff resource. It is because of their personal and professional knowledge of patient care, their ability to interpret research, and their understanding of the challenges bedside nurses must address on a daily basis that make the DNP a future-focused and valued member of a health care team.

A strong clinical background assists in translating research findings into realistic evidence-based practices that nurses can readily incorporate into their daily routines. The CARES tool is an example of this process. The research and literature available on communication and care of the dying and their families are extensive, but application of this research is not occurring in daily nursing practice. Nurses have the basic skills to effectively care for the dying, but they do not possess awareness of the importance of their presence, their compassion, and their humanity. Communication skills were taught in nursing school, but the need to excel at communicating was never emphasized. The CARES tool can only be successfully utilized if good communication exists that allows the nurse to be a strong advocate for the dying individual in their care. The nurse should be the one to ensure all caregivers are acting in unison and focused on the established goals of care.

A method was needed to help nurses improve communication skills, recognize the importance of "just being" and not continually doing, and to anticipate the needs of the dying. Nurses needed to learn what resources were available to meet the specific needs of the dying and how to promote a peaceful death. The CARES tool attempts to give some sense of order and structure to the care of the dying. A sense of urgency and importance is encouraged through reframing the active dying of an individual as an acute event. It is this very same sense of urgency that will be needed to drive this change in nursing practice.

This change in nursing practice to recognize the active dying of an individual as an acute event would require adjustments in staffing to allow a nurse to be present and more available to both the family and the dying individual under his or her care. It could also eliminate the perceived abandonment issues that can occur for the dying and for health care professionals attempting to provide quality end-of-life (EOL) care.

The CARES tool is based on the immense educational resources provided by experts from the End-of-Life National Education Consortium (ELNEC), the National Consensus Project for Quality Palliative Care, and from evidence-based literature reviews. It provides a condensed group of suggestions for the nurse in a format that is easily recalled and applicable to providing compassionate and skillful EOL care. This translation of research findings and evidence-based literature to recommend EOL care that is easily achieved and individualized is the very focus of a DNP.

Clinical competency and the ability to translate research to practice complement the extensive skills of the research-focused PhD. The two doctorate degrees are in a unique position to complement and support each other in the effort to continue to improve care for the dying.

The development and validation plans for the CARES tool are a working example of how PhD-prepared nursing researchers can assist in a DNP translational project. The CARES tool had obtained content and face validity as part of its development, but lacked clinical and statistical validity. A research project was planned, but it soon became apparent that a proposed mixed method research design utilizing pre- and post-testing around a 4-hour orientation and training lecture on the CARES tool, and the collection of responses from a post-analysis focus group, lacked a desired rigor identified by the required institutional review board (IRB) for approval.

The nursing researchers agreed to assist in obtaining IRB approval and identified a need to more clearly differentiate between a quality improvement project, an educational intervention, and a formal research project. The CARES tool was designated as an educational intervention.

A proposal to incorporate clinical and statistical validation of the CARES tool with a house-wide education initiative to instruct nurses on evidence-based care of the dying was developed. This collaboration recognized a need to improve the identification of IRB exempt projects and to expedite the approval process for education and training initiatives house-wide. The entire experience with the IRB is yet another example of the unique contributions that can be made by a DNP functioning within nursing education. The DNP can truly be an agent of change.

As a change agent, the CARES tool was introduced as a poster presentation and as a PowerPoint presentation at various conferences. Permission was granted for numerous requests to reproduce and utilize the CARES tool at several medical institutions in the United States, Canada, and New Zealand. It was a highlighted conference for the week at this author's facility, and efforts are continuing to structure a house-wide training program for nursing staff.

The broad acceptance of the CARES tool led to a book contract with Springer Publishing and collaboration efforts from palliative care focused nursing administrators at Sunnybrook Health Sciences Centre in Toronto, Canada. Sunnybrook has embraced the use of the CARES tool and incorporated its use into their house-wide initiatives to improve care of the dying.

A random audit of deaths occurring at this author's facility from February 2012 to February 2013 was conducted. The audit showed 206 individuals died during the review period, 53% ($n = 109$) died in the intensive care unit (ICU), and 18% ($n = 37$) died on a general oncology unit. These two nursing units would be the first to have their staff receive the planned EOL education. Two additional groups would be included in the first education sessions: the advanced practice nurses working at the facility and the nurses working in pediatrics. Although the pediatric oncology unit only cared for 3% ($n = 6$) of the deaths from the survey, their nursing staff has consistently expressed an interest in learning how to improve their care of the dying. The data collected does not reflect the individuals sent home on hospice and those with whom the staff remained involved through their dying process at home. Many of the pediatric oncology nurses developed close personal bonds with the children they cared for and their families and wanted to improve their skills.

With the initial nursing education group identified, the future educational intervention focused on possible data collection. Two data collection tools were suggested for development. The tools would focus on behavioral changes. One tool would be based on CARES tool content, and a 10-point scale ranging from comfortable to uncomfortable would be utilized to answer questions focused on behaviors and perceived skill. The second tool would be a version of an existing nursing empowerment measurement tool to be reworked to focus on advocacy skills when caring for the dying and their families. Both tools will undergo peer review and validation.

The 4-hour lecture would be based on the ELNEC program modules for symptom management, communication, and the active dying phase. Reference to the CARES tool would be provided throughout the lecture with an emphasis of its full application provided with the discussion on care of the actively dying.

A 6-month trial period is anticipated to allow for the education intervention participants an opportunity to utilize the CARES tool as a guide to influence their care for the dying and their families. After 6 months, 10 study participants would be randomly selected for a focus group discussion on the CARES tool. The questions to be asked would include:

1. Did you find the CARES tool useful?
2. What did you dislike about the CARES tool?
3. What would you like to share about the use of CARES tool?

The PhD-prepared nursing researchers agreed to assist with data collection and analysis to make this planned educational intervention a truly collaborative effort. The plan previously discussed will be given as part of a presentation to nursing administration in an effort to seek approval for a house-wide EOL education program utilizing the CARES tool and to demonstrate the value of a DNP.

Literature review for the CARES tool recognized the need for education, experience, and self-awareness as a primary focus to improve the delivery of EOL care. The CARES tool assists in making education previously provided on care of the dying more specific and easily understood for the bedside nurse and health care provider. It emphasizes the importance of communication and the need to educate families to provide an ability to differentiate a normal dying process from suffering.

The most common needs of the dying are addressed in an acronym format to prompt the health care provider on possible treatments and support to consider. Basic care options address the holistic management of pain, dyspnea, and delirium; promote communication; and provide insight into ethical concerns associated with the delivery of care.

As discussed earlier, additional education on care of the dying is essential and can be obtained by such programs as the ELNEC, developed by the AACN, Washington, DC, and the City of Hope National Medical Center, Los Angeles, California. The program is currently responsible for training 390,000 nurses and health care providers worldwide on care of the dying, representing all 50 states and 77 countries (AACN & COH, 2013). Additional complementary resources include the Association of

Death Education and Counseling (ADEC), and the review of the *Clinical Practice Guidelines for Quality Palliative Care* (3rd edition), developed by the National Consensus Project for Quality Palliative Care (NCP, 2013).

It is important to assess the knowledge level of the nursing groups to be educated on the CARES tool. If minimal education on care of the dying is identified, a foundation in an established education program may be of greatest benefit. Providing the ELNEC program could be the best method for introducing the CARES tool. Only through education can the concepts and suggestions found in the CARES tool be fully understood.

Failures of other pathways and protocols for care of the dying were examined as part of the literature review for the development of the CARES tool. The Liverpool Care of the Dying Pathway (LCP) is perhaps the best example of a failed protocol because the health care providers utilizing the protocol were not adequately educated and trained to understand the correct applications of the pathway. The LCP was developed in the United Kingdom and was once the gold standard for the care of the dying. It was translated into several languages and is utilized throughout Europe and Australia. The LCP was abolished in Great Britain in 2013 following a government review of greater than 600 complaints of neglect. It was concluded that the hospital staff wrongly interpreted the pathway and overmedicated and deprived dying individuals of food and water (Boseley, 2013).

Correct implementation of a pathway or guide is dependent upon the understanding and competency of the health care provider. Often pathways are implemented by individuals with no knowledge base in the disease or condition being addressed.

When attempting to bring research and current evidence-based practice effectively to the bedside, plans to educate must be included. The CARES tool is a translational project that must acknowledge the lessons to be learned from the LCP and encourage education and training in the care of the dying for any health care provider planning to utilize the CARES tool.

Communication and family-driven care is a primary focus of the CARES tool. This emphasis was lacking with the implementation of the LCP, and it is doubtful the omissions in care would have occurred if communication between all involved parties was present, a clear understanding of goals of care was obtained, and there was consistent family involvement regarding decisions of care. The CARES tool is founded on the need for effective communication and in-depth education.

Change requires the presence and direct involvement of experts to ensure understanding and skill levels of the newly trained. The role of the DNP will be essential in maintaining this standard for implementation of the CARES tool.

REFERENCES

American Association of Colleges of Nursing (AACN) & City of Hope National Medical Center (COH). (2013). *ELNEC fact sheet*. Retrieved from http://www.aacn.nche.edu/elnec/about/fact-sheet

Boland, B. A., Treston, J., & O'Sullivan, A. L. (2010). Climb to new educational heights. *The Nurse Practitioner, 35* (4), 36–41.

Boseley, S. (2013). Liverpool care pathway for dying patients to be abolished after review. Retrieved from *The Guardian*. Online [U.S. version]. Retrieved from http://www.theguardian.com/society/2013/jul/15/liverpool-care-pathway-independent-review

NCP. (2013). *Clinical practice guidelines for quality palliative care*. Pittsburgh, PA: National Consensus Project for Quality Palliative Care.

PART V

Additional Applications

CHAPTER 19

A Nursing Model for Care of the Dying

The components of the CARES tool can provide a basis for a nursing care model specific to the care of the dying, their families, and for individuals who provide care for the dying. The major concepts identified in the CARES tool can be diagrammed to allow for a more holistic focus on the unique needs of the dying (see Figure 19.1).

The CARES tool model places the dying and their families at the center. Their needs are the focus of all care provided. There are three immediate subgroups that address the most common needs and/or issues when caring for the dying. The three subgroups are symptom management, emotional and spiritual care, and self-care.

SYMPTOM MANAGEMENT

Symptom management is divided into the three most common symptom management needs of the dying and their families found in peer-reviewed literature, and include comfort, airway, and restlessness and delirium. The first category is comfort.

Comfort

Comfort has four areas to be addressed:

1. Pain
2. Comfort measures
3. Education
4. Communication

FIGURE 19.1 The CARES tool model of nursing care for the dying.

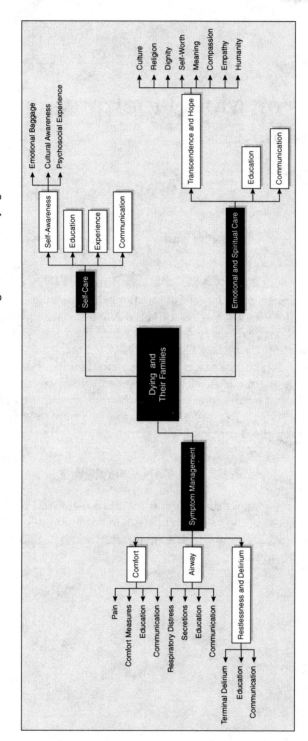

The need for a dying patient to have their pain under control and not to suffer physically or psychosocially is crucial to achieving a peaceful death. A dying patient only has minimal energy. If patients must use this energy to overcome physical or emotional distress they will be unable to focus on the spiritual needs of closure, establishing meaning, legacy building, and preparing their families for a life without them.

Nurses can monitor closely for pain and infer pain is present if they note increased restlessness, increased heart rate, diaphoresis, moaning, or changes from baseline behaviors, which the family may note and feel are pain responses unique to the individual. It is important to include family members in the assessment of an unconscious patient's pain level. The family knows this person and can more readily detect signs of pain. At the very least, it helps family members to feel involved in their loved one's care. The nurse must keep in mind the research evidence that concluded that, if an individual is in pain before becoming unresponsive, he or she is likely to remain in pain. Withdrawal of pain medication to assess responsiveness in a dying patient is cruel. The risks do not outweigh the benefits, and the only persons being cared for are often the care providers concerned with legal implications of the use of opioids. We are now seeing health care providers being successfully sued for not providing adequate pain management. Assessment and an ethical approach to pain management are essential.

Nurses caring for the dying individual play an important role in the promotion of comfort. They can limit unnecessary blood draws and procedures and encourage as much time as possible for the dying to spend time with their families.

Education is important for care providers as they must understand basic pain management physiology and methods to control pain. This needed education is beyond the scope of the CARES tool. Education is a component of all the subgroups in the CARES tool model to emphasize the need for the nurse to seek additional training and knowledge about the care of the dying. With education comes understanding and an ability to embrace the importance and supportive research that needs to be reflected in the care of the dying.

Communication is also listed as a component of each subgroup in the CARES tool model. Communication and compassion are the very foundation of the CARES tool. Without them, the CARES tool would function like any other reference or protocol. Care of the dying requires a unique set of skills centered on our very humanity. Our ability to advocate for the persons under our care and their families is dependent upon the clear understanding of their goals of care. Establishing goals of care requires the dying and their families' ability to make informed decisions. Informed decisions can only be made if we openly communicate and compassionately provide information according to confirmed wishes and boundaries set by the dying individual and his or her family. Without effective lines of communication, nurses cannot function as fully supportive advocates promoting the peaceful death for individuals under their care. Communication is addressed in more depth in Chapter 15.

Airway Management

Airway management is the next subgroup of symptom management in the CARES tool model. There are four components of the airway subgroup:

1. Respiratory distress
2. Secretions
3. Education
4. Communication

Respiratory distress or dyspnea is a common result of the dying process and there are effective measures that can be taken to reduce the perception of shortness of breath and feelings of suffocation. As stated in previous chapters, the use of morphine remains the gold standard of care. It reduces the workload of the heart by improving myocardial perfusion through coronary dilatation and reduces preload. No effort is made to speed the dying process; the focus is rather on reducing suffering. Providing clear explanations of treatments and procedures will help family members be more comfortable with the care provided to their loved one. One of the most important goals of symptom management for the dying is to educate the family on the difference between a normal physical response in the dying process and suffering.

Dyspnea provides one of the clearest examples of the need to differentiate between the normal dying process and suffering. As the dying individual progresses, the brain receives less oxygen due to reduced vascular circulation. Breathing is completely involuntary and fully controlled by the brain stem as the loss of all respiratory stimulation mechanisms continue to fail. The result is often an irregular agonal respiration that can be interpreted as a gasping-like effort. Accessory muscles may be involved and can produce a flailing-like chest motion in a final effort by the body to pull in oxygen. The result can be very difficult for a family member to watch and it is at this time the nurse is needed most to provide reassurance and to explain what is occurring.

Family members may request additional oxygen be provided. If the nurse explores risks versus benefits of this action, he or she could explain that the additional oxygen:

1. Will not stop the dying process but could make the dying individual's body take longer to die, and increase any associated physical suffering

2. Could make any last communication more difficult

3. Cannot be utilized by the body at this terminal stage and will not stop the observed agonal breathing

If family members continue to express discomfort over the final breathing efforts of their loved one, it is reasonable to provide oxygen through a nasal cannula at 2 L/min. This amount of oxygen should not add or detract from the dying process and is a perfect example of the point at which the nurse must shift his or her focus to caring for the family. They are the ones who will need to live with the memory of their loved one suffering, whether or not their perception is based on fact. If providing additional oxygen helps comfort the family, it should be offered.

The second area of consideration when addressing airway function symptom management is the increase in pooling oropharyngeal secretions. Management is commonly centered on the use of anticholinergics. Suctioning is an additional option that may actually stimulate more secretions but can provide the family a last loving task and promote a feeling of usefulness in them. This is but one more situation the nurse must evaluate risks versus benefits and advocate for the greatest comfort for the individuals under his or her care. Suctioning may not alter the workload of breathing for the dying, but it will help to reduce the family's anxiety.

Education as discussed earlier remains invaluable for the care provider to be comfortable with the management of respiration issues of the dying. There must be an ongoing teaching of the family to explain your actions and to help them understand the comfort measures being utilized.

Communication that is clear, supportive, and compassionate will help the family adjust and correctly differentiate a normal dying course from suffering. Again, effective, sincere, and empathetic communication must be utilized. The nurse should continue to act by weighing the risks versus the benefits of his or her actions for the dying individual while acknowledging the concerns of the family.

Restlessness and Delirium

Restlessness and delirium is the final subgroup of symptom management. It includes the need to address:

1. Terminal delirium

2. Education

3. Communication

Terminal delirium, as described in detail in Chapter 9, is a common condition requiring skilled end-of-life symptom management for 80% of the dying population. There are some common causes such as pain and a distended bladder that can be quickly remedied; however, causes such as urinary tract infections may require further discussion before treating. Goals of care should be reviewed before starting antibiotics, especially if the delirium is controllable with antipsychotics or benzodiazepines.

Managing terminal delirium like the other previously discussed common symptom management needs of the dying requires a clear understanding of the physiology of dying, education to understand options of care, and strong communication skills to clearly convey the risks versus the benefits of treating possible causes of terminal delirium. All the components of the restlessness and delirium subgroup require effective interaction to manage. There may be a need to treat the root cause of the delirium if it can be identified, educate the family on options of care, and clearly communicate that the effects of treatment may further reduce any meaningful interaction with their loved one. This can be a difficult time for families as it may be the first separation they encounter from their loved one, making death much more of a reality. The family will rely on the nurse for guidance and support as the individual they love can no longer communicate with them.

EMOTIONAL AND SPIRITUAL CARE

Emotional and spiritual care is the second subgroup of the CARES tool model for care of the dying and their families. It is composed of three major divisions:

1. Transcendence and hope
2. Education
3. Communication

The division transcendence and hope is further divided into the concepts of culture, religion, dignity, self-worth, meaning, compassion, empathy, and humanity. All components play a role in sustaining the spiritual need to feel valued and respected. It is only in this type of environment that both goal-based hope (GBh) and emotion-based hope (EBh) can survive and allow for the transcendence of fears and anxieties necessary to achieve a peaceful death (see Chapter 2).

As in all subgroups of the CARES tool model, an emphasis on education and communication is again encouraged. Knowledge gained on spirituality, hope, and transcendence and the ability to share this knowledge and to communicate it effectively are the best methods of holistic support the caregiver can provide the dying and their families.

SELF-CARE

Self-care is the final subgroup to be discussed in the CARES tool model. It is composed of:

1. Self-awareness
2. Education
3. Experience
4. Communication

Self-care is necessary for the caregiver in both the professional health care and family provider setting. Self-awareness dictates that care providers be aware of their personal energy resources and seek any necessary support so they can continue to be of service to the dying. Too often burnout, emotional distress, and fatigue, both emotional and physical, can occur. Caregivers must be self-aware of their personal needs and care for themselves so that they can continue to care for others.

Self-awareness can be achieved through education, experience, and effective communication. The need to be supported by one's peers is basic to our human nature. We all have a need to be appreciated, honored, and cared about. Being self-aware allows us to seek out the support we require and to acknowledge our own biases that may interfere with providing quality end-of-life care.

A nurse that experienced a traumatic and unsupported death may hesitate to take an assignment to care for a dying individual and his or her family. Another nurse may simply lack any experience caring for the dying and may accept the assignment but decide to minimize his or her availability. In both cases, self-awareness is essential. If a nurse is self-aware, he or she can consciously choose the behaviors they wish to provide. Caring for the dying is not the time to be frightened or feel forced to support and communicate with individuals under your care. Interactions should be genuine, compassionate, and empathetic. Forced and automated actions will be recognized by the individuals under your care and often decisions are made to not seek your assistance. This can lead to feelings of abandonment and complicated grieving for families and for the dying.

Nurses must be self-aware of the talents and gifts they possess that can help an individual and their family through the dying process. They must recognize their personal barriers and seek out other health care professionals to fill the gaps in care or to fully take over. Being a strong advocate for individuals may mean you recognize that your skill sets do not match the requirements needed for care, and you will need to find someone who can take over.

Self-awareness also requires the nurse to become aware of his or her own symptoms of overidentification, grief, secondary stress, emotional exhaustion, and/or growing depression and emotional fatigue. We must embrace our responsibility to seek help to resolve or at least modify these issues so that the care provided to the terminally ill is not compromised. Help can be available through group support and the verbalizing of feelings as described in Chapter 12.

The need for continuing education and improving communication skills is again emphasized. The importance of nurses to accept they are human and can professionally grieve and assist other professionals in their grieving process is both free and humble. Learning more about this process and sharing our findings with our coworkers will greatly assist nurses in becoming emotionally stronger so that they can continue to address the many challenges of caring for the dying.

Research studies have noted that the nurses with the best communication and self-care skills were those with the most experience in caring for the dying (Murray-Frommelt, 1991). Experience provides practice of skills and increases self-confidence allowing for genuine and empathetic communication and interactions.

All subgroups emphasize the need for education to improve knowledge and understanding and good communication skills to successfully address the specific requirements of the dying. No one subgroup is more important than the other. They are all independent needs and they all must be present and functional at the same time to provide quality care for the dying and their families.

The CARES tool model provides a graphic demonstration of the components of the CARES tool and what is needed to provide quality evidence-based care for the dying. The emphasis for further education on care of the dying is evident in all categories. It is a prerequisite for effective communication and advocacy. Ongoing education should be a yearly staff improvement goal.

REFERENCE

Murray-Frommelt, K. H. (1991). The effects of death education on nurses' attitudes toward caring for terminally ill persons and their families. *American Journal of Hospice and Palliative Medicine, 8*(5), 37–43.

CHAPTER 20

Versions and Influence of the CARES Tool

Additional support programs, tools, and professional attitude changes have evolved because of the impact of the CARES tool on health care staff. This has resulted in the establishment of nursing-focused grieving rounds to identify and suggest methods to address and possibly reconcile issues of professional grieving, secondary stress, and burnout; the development of a supportive personnel version of the CARES tool to assist and encourage nonmedical staff involvement in the care of the dying and their families; and a renewed appreciation and advancement of camaraderie between coworkers occurring as a result of learning to effectively care for the dying.

The CARES tool assists in the promotion of individualized care for dying patients and utilizes a stronger focus on spirituality and employing compassion and humanity. This emphasis on humanity and compassion has ultimately influenced the way health care providers interact with each other. The focus on self-care as part of the CARES tool has resulted in the development of a monthly support group meeting held on an intensive care unit (ICU), called grieving rounds. A trial of a 1-hour block of time the last Thursday of every month in the ICU at the City of Hope was scheduled. The format was much like grand rounds when difficult cases are reviewed and constructive criticism and alternative methods to manage care are discussed. In grieving rounds, the nurses in ICU pre-select cases involving the death of patients they found particularly challenging and then planned to discuss them at this designated time.

Grieving rounds was intended to be an open forum to discuss any questions or concerns about the care of a dying individual in the ICU. Nurses often shared their personal feelings of failure and frustration. Professional grief was often explored with the help of a social worker, a psychologist, a spiritual care counselor, and a palliative care nurse practitioner that routinely attend the monthly sessions. Confirmation and support of professional grieving, recognition of secondary traumatic stress syndrome, and issues of compassion fatigue were often identified and discussed. The trial of this program began in January 2013. Twenty ICU nurses have participated over the course of 1 year. When interviewed about the usefulness of the program, participants stated positive results such as feelings of being listened to, valued, and supported. With the routine presence of a social worker, a spiritual counselor, and a palliative care nurse practitioner, nurses obtained needed emotional support and strategies to better cope with the psychosocial and emotional pressures of caring for the dying. Many of the nurses stated they regained emotional strength just knowing the program was available and that their managers cared enough about them to provide the service.

Another creative benefit of providing training for care of the dying utilizing the CARES tool resulted in a type of group therapy. Eight non-nursing hospital employees in the department of supportive care medicine agreed to become involved in a project to improve the understanding of care needed to support a dying individual and his or her family. The group composed of social workers, child-life specialists, receptionists, patient navigators, and psychologists wanted to explore how they could assist nurses and physicians as they cared for the dying. They chose to review the CARES tool and planned to develop a supportive care version for non-nursing/physician staff. Initial review of the CARES tool stimulated participants to openly share their personal stories about the death of someone close to them and their fears and concerns about death and dying. Items in the CARES tool prompted many questions and even more personal stories as the group expressed excitement over the important role they could play in caring for the dying. An openness and shared support evolved within the group. A form of emotional cleansing occurred that seemed to affect every member of the group as they voluntarily shared their personal stories about death and dying. Participants were seen at their most vulnerable, and tears were openly shared with one touching story after another. Ultimately, over the course of a few weeks, the study group became very close and supportive of each other even outside the education sessions. They were able to work effectively to develop the supportive care version of the CARES tool that emphasized the following prompts and suggestions for care of the dying and their families.

▨ Comfort

- Help to minimize or prevent interruptions between the dying and their families from unnecessary procedures and treatment
- Support the family and patient care wishes and assist the nurse with the communication of those wishes
- Assist in the providing of a continuous presence

Airway

- Reinforce explanations given about breathing changes that occur in the dying process to help differentiate them from suffering
- Suggest the use of a fan to help with feelings of shortness of breath and anxiety related to dyspnea
- Be present in room as much as possible to help reassure families and the dying
- Reinforce the comforting effects of touch and use of soft speech

Restlessness and delirium

- Reinforce teaching provided on causes of confusion/delirium
- Encourage providing familiar sounds such as favorite music, smells, and use of touch
- Assist in advocating for the dying and their families by keeping the primary nurse informed and assisting the nurse as possible
- Continue to maintain a reassuring presence, and explain possible causes of behavior changes

Emotional and spiritual support

- Work with the health care providers to supply therapeutic presence, active listening, and restatement of information provided by the primary nurse as needed
- Encourage the family to talk directly to the dying individual, and to emphasize the dying individual's need for reassurance
- Never underestimate the power of a washcloth (any act of kindness and compassion will be remembered and appreciated by the family)
- Assist with desired family rituals, requested activities, and the notification of desired support persons as necessary
- Always maintain a therapeutic presence that conveys compassion, caring, and approachability
- Continue to provide an example of calm and peacefulness

Self-care

- Seek out group support to ventilate concerns and emotional issues
- Acknowledge that professional grieving is normal and seek support of coworkers
- Attend grief support programs as needed
- Acknowledge the very important role you played with the grieving family

The complete digital file for the supportive care personnel version of the CARES tool can be obtained from the City of Hope Pain and Palliative Care Resource site http://prc.coh.org/res_inst.asp or by contacting Bonnie Freeman at bofreeman@coh.org.

Upon completion of the tool, all subcommittee group members ($n = 8$) were asked, "What did you learn from your experience developing the supportive version of the CARES tool?" The group member's responses underwent analysis for common themes. The following six themes were identified.

1. **Validation of emotions/feeling they were not alone:** All group members felt compelled to share their personal and professional stories about death and caring for the dying. At first they struggled with a sense of vulnerability, but soon found group members to be compassionate, understanding, and equally as vulnerable. All members were supportive and empathetic as similar stories of loss, feelings of abandonment, and unresolved grief were shared. The immediate response of the group was to console, and all realized how comforting it was to just have someone listen to their stories. Ultimately, it was acknowledged how much we all had in common and how similar our stories were.

2. **Increased ability to share feelings:** All group members noted how easy it became to share feelings once trust was established based on the common emotional issues identified by group members. This emotional support helped some members find closure and others were able to talk about issues for the first time. When the content of the CARES tool is reviewed, the desire to share personal and professional experience is very common. It is rare to find an outlet for discussions about death and dying, and the group members developing this tool embraced the opportunity. Everyone participated equally and enthusiastically. The courage to talk about death and dying experiences caused supportive and caring friendships to evolve.

3. **Provided ability to process feelings:** The group freely shared their feelings. This dialogue flowed easier with each meeting. It soon became a challenge to stay on task as members wanted to continue sharing experiences and welcomed the advice and emotional support that was so freely given. Many realized there was nothing further they could have done, and one individual was able to let go of her guilt for not being present the very moment her mother died. The supportive version of the CARES tool helped group members understand the difference between a normal dying process and suffering.

4. **Find some control over the uncontrollable:** Group members found putting the emotional baggage they carried into words helped them to finally accept they did all they could regarding the death experiences they shared. Many expressed a wish to have known some of the content of the CARES tool when they were assisting someone through the dying process. The realization of tangible things they could have done both saddened some group members and strengthened the resolve of others to use this knowledge gained when confronted with similar circumstances. Some group members expressed amazement how just their presence could impact a dying individual and his or her family.

5. **Given concrete methods to help families:** The group felt many of the suggested tasks and communication prompts provided them with a variety of actions they could draw from to support the nurse's teachings and comfort the grieving family.

6. **Increased comfort when working with the dying:** It was felt the CARES tool helped to normalize an otherwise panic situation. Group members enjoyed learning what to expect and how to prepare to meet some of the common emotional and spiritual needs of families and the dying. Many members in the group verbalized their surprise at how much they could help, and the difference they could make in the lives of grieving family members.

A final unanticipated effect the project had on group members was the development of a strong emotional bond that formed and resulted in the establishment of deep friendships. This cohesive effect stimulated by discussions prompted from the development of the supportive care version of the CARES tool is still evident with any interaction among group members.

Group members wanted to expand use of the supportive version of the CARES tool as they found the CARES tool to be readily adaptable for use by other members of the health care team. Providing effective evidence-based symptom management and promoting and supporting self-transcendence for the dying and their families through compassion, empathy, and the use of our humanity were identified as universal for any job role that results in contact with the dying and their families.

Obtaining education and experience in care of the dying was found to be essential for anyone desiring to care for the dying. It was identified that primary nurses caring for the dying often need support if they must leave to address related care issues or assess the needs of another individual under their care. If a social worker or dietician happens to be in the room and was trained on the CARES tool, he or she could be prepared to reinforce the nurse's teaching, answer questions, or know how to obtain needed resources to effectively support the dying individual and his or her family.

It was also identified that all persons caring for the dying should be self-aware. All individuals are affected by personal, emotional, cultural, and psychosocial experiences that may negatively alter the support they can provide. It was believed that support should continue to be provided for hospital employees working with the dying, and plans were developed to provide department-specific support group meetings similar to the ones established for the grieving rounds in ICU.

A final suggested use for the CARES tool was to incorporate it with the teaching provided to staff and volunteer personnel participating in the No One Dies Alone (NODA) program. The NODA program (http://www.eskenazihealth.edu/our-services/palliative-care-program/NODA)

was established by Sandra Clarke RN, CCRN, at Peace Health Hospital in Eugene, Oregon, in 2001. The volunteer NODA program was developed in response to Sandra's frustration over the quality of care she provided a dying gentleman. This individual died alone because Sandra was too busy caring for her other assigned patients. Sandra felt there was a need to obtain and train volunteers to sit with the dying individual and allow the family to take breaks, and to provide comfort and companionship when the primary nurse could not remain at the bedside.

A modification to the NODA program was suggested based on the spiritual and communication prompts found in the CARES tool. Plans would include training of all hospital personnel to both the NODA information and the supportive care personnel version of the CARES tool. A basic introduction to the program could be offered as part of general orientation and then hospital staff would be free to volunteer for the in-depth training. Volunteers who complete the NODA/CARES training could notify the nursing house supervisor of their availability if needed to sit with a dying patient. This plan could ensure available staff during the off shifts and through the night, often the most difficult time for volunteer availability and the most common time for dying to occur. The use of trained volunteers could greatly assist the primary nurse caring for the dying patient and his or her family. Their presence would also ensure a hospital staff person's continuous presence to support and comfort the dying.

Providing basic information about a care of the dying volunteer program for all hospital staff could:

1. Enable individuals who decide not to volunteer to possess a basic understanding of what other volunteers are doing and to more readily agree to provide coverage for their responsibilities if necessary.

2. Assist in meeting the general staff education requirements for palliative care certification through JCAHO.

3. Provide evidence of interdepartmental collaboration to meet a recognized patient care need for Magnet status application.

4. Assist with the education needs of all staff regarding the unique requirements of the dying and their families.

5. Encourage personal review of death and dying, and possibly stimulate family discussions and completion of advance directives for hospital personnel.

The various creative uses of the CARES tool prompted a desire to extend the emphasized use of communication and compassion to fellow coworkers and not just the individuals under their care. There was a common desire to openly and freely share personal experiences and feelings about death. Tears and laughter would flow freely, and a sense of a shared vulnerability allowed for compassionate listening and genuine caring and support.

Health care providers obtained firsthand experience of the important role our compassion and empathy plays when attempting to assist the dying and their families. This was a small example of what the health care provider gained when learning how to care for the dying and their families. Wicks (2012) explains this phenomenon in *Riding the Dragon*:

> When all of life—both the perceived "good" and "bad"—is faced directly with a sense of openness, life's promises are more fully realized. Moreover, this is not only important for the person's experiencing the struggles but also for those they may touch after absorbing the new lessons learned about gratitude, impermanence/the fragility of life, simplicity, meaning-making, and compassion. (p. ii.)

REFERENCE

Wicks, R. J. (2012). *Riding the dragon: Ten lessons for inner strength in challenging times.* Notre Dame, IN: Sorin Books.

CHAPTER 21

Preserving Hope

Many of the dying do not fear death as much as they fear how they will die (Byock, 2012). Prolonged suffering remains common and can result in feelings of hopelessness, which encompasses much more than just physical pain. It can occur with any sense of loss or feelings of vulnerability (Byock, 2012; Coward, 2010). Suffering is subjective and can include actual or perceived emotional, physical, social, or spiritual distress. It is a common response among the dying with or without actual physical pain (Coward & Reed, 1996; Ersek, 2006). It can range from feelings of uneasiness to excruciating torment as the individual struggles to accept the loss of previous life roles and independence (Byock, 1997; Ersek, 2006; Longaker, 1998).

A primary role of nurses and the palliative care team caring for the terminally ill is to address this suffering and provide hope. Yet, the medical community still views the decision to consult palliative care as an acknowledgment that all hope is lost and the terminally ill will surrender to their disease and die. The involvement of palliative care teams becomes a double-edged sword: There is the belief that providing palliative care will add to the comfort and quality of an individual's life, but the price to be paid is the acknowledgment that the individual is dying. Avoidance of reality now becomes a strong and often a subconscious collaborator in the medical management of the terminally ill.

Education is essential to help the medical community understand the hope that can be obtained through the involvement of a palliative care interdisciplinary team. This knowledge deficit presents one of the greatest hurdles to consulting palliative care early and avoiding the chaos of last-minute panic and grief that can occur when a family and the health care staff are unprepared to support the actively dying.

The CARES tool was designed to help bridge this gap in care. Nurses are made aware of what orders they should obtain and are provided suggestions on communication and comfort measures they can provide within their scope of practice. Much of end-of-life (EOL) care can be nurse driven and does not require a formal diagnosis of dying to initiate. Nurses can request consults for members of the palliative care team without calling it a palliative care consult. Often, this is argued as just merely semantics, but the process seems to be more acceptable when the physician is asked for individual consults for spiritual care, social work, and pain management. The choice to move toward EOL care is difficult to accept all at once. It is more easily taken on in small doses. This holds true not only for the dying and their families, but also for health care providers (HCPs).

As human beings we all face our share of loss and overwhelming stress, so the ability to over identify with the dying and their families can be strong. If small steps are taken toward supporting the needs of the dying rather than denying them, or aggressively confronting the issue by demanding physicians acknowledge the individual under their care is dying, much can be accomplished. Robert Wicks (2012) in his book *Riding the Dragon: Ten Lessons for Inner Strength in Challenging Times* notes if one can take adversity in small doses, be open and flexible, in other words "ride our dragons," so much more can be accomplished than through the use of denial or direct confrontation. Wicks (2012) observed this method of goal achievement can be transforming. It allows all parties involved to adjust to the dying process and the eventual death of another human being.

Nurses could request a palliative care consult when they feel their measures are not effective, or they want additional support in meeting the needs of the individuals under their care. By this time, the seeds of acceptance have been planted and open consulting and involvement of a palliative care team may be possible.

The hesitancy for physicians to consult palliative care is a cultural bias that must be addressed to ensure that the best possible quality care can be provided to all patients in this country. A stigma exists that implies the presence of palliative care staff means a patient is now without hope and must be near death. This is due largely to the direct association of palliative care with hospice. Palliative care plays an extensive role for the dying and their families, but it has a role in any illness or disease process. Palliative care is simply comfort care and symptom management. It applies to anyone healthy or ill. A greater acceptance has occurred when the palliative care interdisciplinary team is consulted for pain management, but still there is a concern of undue influence on patients to "give up." Often, medical personnel believe a consult to palliative care implies incompetency, failure, and an inability to provide for the emotional needs of their patients and families rather than a source for additional resources and support. It is believed only a curative mode of care can provide hope.

A shift to a comfort focus in care can imply that all hope is lost and it is time for the palliative care interdisciplinary team to take over. It is common to hear physicians and staff members say, "I don't want to consult palliative care because my patient is not that sick," or "I am not ready to give up hope." The primary reason palliative care is associated only with death and loss of hope is that they are often consulted too late in the disease process.

Palliative care cannot only preserve but promote and encourage hope by helping the dying and their families "ride the dragon" and confront their fears and concerns about suffering, promote effective communication, and find closure.

> In the darkness, if we are open to seeing our helplessness and facing our loss and trauma directly, the result will be to experience the cardinal psychological and spiritual virtue of humility. When this occurs, wondrous results become possible; because when you take humility and add to it knowledge, you get wisdom. And when you add this gift of wisdom to compassion, you are in a position to offer selfless love. What more can you ask for than that? (Wicks, 2012, p. ii)

This quote from Robert Wicks is intended as much for the dying individual and his or her family as it is for health care personnel. There is a need to provide what is best and most needed for persons under our care and their families and not what is comfortable and flattering of our skills. Hope is not stagnant. It is more than a goal; it is also a feeling of security, acceptance, and a belief in one's ability to transcend adversity.

Hope is a basic human need. C. Fanslow-Brunjes (2008) noted, "There is no such thing as a person without some type of hope. No one can live or die for even a moment without hope." Hope is associated with faith, love, and charity and is considered one of the essential attributes of Christianity. The concept of hope has been around for centuries. It was hope that remained in Pandora's box after it was opened and all worldly evils and sufferings were released upon humankind.

Hope can be both simple and very complex. When analyzed in depth the spiritual focus of hope is often diluted as we struggle to fully define this concept, but it is that indefinable spiritual strength that makes hope so important. To fully understand the many facets of hope, it must be viewed with both the mind and the heart.

The intellectual focus of hope acknowledges this very important human requirement as a specific desire, wish, or goal. This type of hope can best be described as goal-based hope (GBh; Wittenberg-Lyles, Goldsmith, & Ragan, 2011). But, hope is so much more; it is also a nonspecific and intangible emotion or sense. The heart's view of hope is one of optimism; it views life as a wealth of possibilities. Hope is characterized as a sense or a feeling, such as a feeling of hopefulness. This sense or nonspecific feeling requires a positive personal perception of one's own dignity, self-worth, and a positive view of the future in the face of hardship, sadness, disease, and misfortune. This internalized, heartfelt sense of hope can be identified as emotion-based hope (EBh). It is difficult if not impossible for one form of hope to exist without the presence of the other. In illness the wish, desire, or prayer for a cure is GBh. It is often the most dominant form of hope, but the energy and focus to sustain GBh must be supported by EBh obtained through spiritual and emotional support that clearly validates the worthiness of the individual, and confirms that he or she is so much more than the disease. GBh is related to explicit outcomes; EBh is the emotional and spiritual energy that allows us to believe our goals, desires, or wishes are possible.

Hope, both GB and EB, does not end with a terminal diagnosis or with a pronouncement of futility. The dominant form of hope in a terminal situation often becomes emotion-based. Hope becomes a process toward a sense of peace, safety, and acceptance if it is allowed to evolve through open communication, symptom management, and emotional and spiritual support (Wittenberg-Lyles et al., 2011). EBh plays an important role as comfort becomes the focus of care. It must be nurtured through respect, autonomy, empathy, and dignity as patients, families, and medical staff prepare to face new challenges that address quality of life and EOL care. EBh can fuel a sense of closure, emotional and spiritual peace, and feelings of safety if allowed to evolve. It supports the development of new GBh such as hope for new treatments, hope to prolong life, and hope for a peaceful death (Fanslow-Brunjes, 2008).

Hope has been with humankind for centuries. It has become a common word in our vocabulary, and for many, GBh is the only known definition of hope.

The frequent misuse of the word *hope* does not diminish the presence of EBh, especially, when it so accurately describes the inner processes and emotional strength it can provide the chronically and terminally ill. Hope can and must exist throughout the human life cycle, even in death (Duggleby, 2001).

GBh for a cure is a common emotion as an individual and his or her family face the challenges of an illness. It reflects the curative focus of medical care in our "forever young and healthy" culture (Wittenberg-Lyles et al., 2011). Medical technology has advanced dramatically to support our belief of immortality, and now even cancer is considered a chronic disease. Modern medicine may not be able to cure a chronic disease completely but it can slow the progression and attempt to control side effects and complications related to the disease process and treatment. EBh provides the emotional strength to fight the disease and wait for a possible cure. For over 90 million people in this country with chronic diseases like cancer, diabetes, chronic obstructive pulmonary disease (COPD), and congestive heart failure (CHF), the "wait" could span 20 to 40 years. There is a need for skillful symptom management, support for overwhelmed primary caregivers, and promotion of a desired quality of life uniquely defined by the individual and his or her family before any focus of EOL issues are addressed. Both GBh and EBh play an important role in any illness.

Hope is essential to all human beings; it is strongly associated with our ability to cope and to challenge our fate. Both GBh and EBh cannot fully evolve in the presence of suffering, nor can it be nurtured by HCPs that view an individual's needs and goals as foolish or futile (Groopman, 2004). Hope is uniquely defined by the individual and his or her family. It can become a possibility of a future free of pain and suffering. It represents an inner process of courage and emotional strength to endure, and to preserve one's quality of life and dignity. Hope may seem contradictory when addressing suffering, and the chronically and terminally ill. EBh actually flourishes with aggressive symptom management and skillful spiritual and emotional support (Ersek & Cotter, 2010).

It is the responsibility of HCPs to identify, respect, and nurture an individual and the family's hopes. The palliative care team strives to assist the HCP and most specifically the bedside nurse, to this end. They can provide teaching, training, support, and consultants that will help to nurture a terminally ill individual and the family's hopes. Ultimately, hope is all any of us really have.

The palliative care interdisciplinary team provides an extensive resource of social workers, chaplains, nurse liaisons, educators, pharmacists, case managers, physicians, nurse practitioners, and volunteers all working together to provide for the physical, spiritual, psychological, social, and emotional needs of our ever growing patient population. They can address challenges of prolonged chronic illness through strong partnerships with primary physicians, nurses, patients, families, community, and other HCPs. The control of chronic symptoms such as pain, fatigue, depression, nausea, constipation, delirium, anxiety, and dyspnea is possible with knowledgeable, aggressive management. When chronic symptoms are controlled patients and families can retain some quality of life and continue to hope as they define it. Common hopes include GBh such as hope for a future free of pain, hope for a return to a life of quality, hope for a cure, hope for more time, and EBh for a sense of peace. Palliative care's focus and ultimate goal is to nurture and support our patients and the families' hopes.

When GBh and EBh combine, a patient's hope is more profound than a just a wish or a goal. It evolves into a desire to achieve a perceived need that is believed to be possible and significant to the individual. Hope is a method of coping that can provide a sense of control over the uncontrollable (Ersek & Cotter, 2010). To hope is to believe in the ability to control circumstances and to no longer be at the mercy of outside forces (Groopman, 2004). Hope provides motivation, strength, and the will to challenge life or to prepare for eventual death. Hope is strongly associated with coping (Ersek & Cotter, 2010). Hope directly influences health and adaptation to illness. Patients and their families' desire to hope can be supported physically, spiritually, socially, psychologically, and emotionally with the assistance and resources of the palliative care team.

The palliative care interdisciplinary team provides the following resources:

1. Social workers to help reduce stress through education and supplying resources that can address patient and family issues/concerns to allow more time to focus on emotional, physical, and spiritual healing. They provide psychosocial supportive counseling, and referrals for any identified needs. Many institutions turn to their social workers to also assist with bed placement and discharge planning.

2. RN liaisons or navigators work to ensure communication by providing personalized guidance, support, and assistance to individuals and their families. They are made aware of appointments and schedules and help negotiate the complex health care system to allow for consistent, quality care.

3. MD and NPs provide direct assessment and medical management of symptoms that will calm and comfort chronic and terminally ill individuals and their families and promote quality of life.

4. Psychiatrists provide expertise to identify and address emotional and psychological issues the patient and family may be addressing. They are instrumental in the treatment of depression, delirium, and the emotional concerns of our patients.

5. Pharmacists provide recommendations, education, and support of patients, families, and staff to understand and utilize the best pharmaceutical treatment possible that is in keeping with patient- and family-identified goals.

6. Nutritionists offer teaching and guidance to meet the patient's specific nutritional needs, and provide expertise through suggestions and recommendations.

7. Case managers provide communication with outside resources to meet the needs of the individual and his or her family. They interact with hospice and other agencies to expedite plans of care and to promote quality of life.

8. Spiritual counselors provide understanding and support for all faiths and coordinate spiritual care with specific denominations and religious leaders.

9. Volunteers are an essential part of the palliative care team. They are involved in fund raising, and directly supporting our patients and families through companionship, listening, acting as resource guides, providing directions, and reassurance.

10. Others such as music therapists, acupuncturists, aromatherapists, meditation experts, and art therapists, all work to provide nonpharmaceutical comfort and emotional, spiritual, and psychological support. This category could also include occupational therapists, physical therapists, recreational therapists, and speech and language pathologists.

The palliative care interdisciplinary team works to provide specific support needed for each individual and family member under their care as they work through illness and resolve the sense of suffering.

As stated earlier, hope cannot evolve and be sustained in the presence of suffering. Suffering encompasses much more than physical perceptions of pain. It can occur with any sense of loss or feelings of vulnerability. "Suffering is experienced by people, not bodily organs. That which threatens the wholeness or the survival of the person results in suffering" (Ersek & Cotter, 2010).

> Suffering comes from our aversion and resistance to our painful circumstances, not from the pain itself. Suffering is our agony at losing our hopes and expectations, being forced to relinquish control, and feeling vulnerable and powerless against the undesired change or loss. (Longaker, 1998, p. 48)

Suffering is subjective and can include any actual or perceived emotional, physical, social, or spiritual distress. It is a common response among the chronically ill and dying with or without actual physical pain. It can range from feelings of uneasiness to excruciating torment as the individual struggles to accept the loss of previous life roles and independence. "Existence that is merely a burden and lacks a future with any direction or point produces the worst kind of suffering" (Byock, 1997, p. 83). The palliative care interdisciplinary team acknowledges the suffering of the individual and his or her family and can lessen the emotional burdens through empathy, active listening, dignity affirming therapies, and demonstrating and promoting respect for them as individuals and unique human beings. Spiritual counselors, social workers, and psychiatrists can work with patients and families to address their suffering and arrive at more peaceful resolutions. This kind of support should occur early in the disease process to allow time for physical, emotional, psychological, and/ or spiritual healing and possibly resolution. Suffering is not exclusive to the actively dying.

Hope is nurtured when pain and suffering are diminished, caring relationships are supported, and faith and spirituality are enhanced. Uncontrolled pain and suffering greatly contributes to a sense of hopelessness and results in "overwhelming fatigue and lack of energy to invest in the hoping process" (Duggleby, 2001, p. 53). The palliative care interdisciplinary team considers pain and symptom management the cornerstone of their program. Hope requires energy and focus that is often depleted or diverted when an individual is in pain. Pain, like suffering, is not always physical. Pain can be emotional, psychological, and spiritual. Palliative care can assist in identifying sources of pain and suffering and effectively address individual and family needs to allow for hope to survive.

Caring relationships foster EBh through the willingness of the participants to share a part of themselves, listen attentively, and provide an emotional escape through reminiscing, humor, and laughter. The palliative care interdisciplinary team can provide the emotional, spiritual, and psychological support and encouragement so difficult to make available by the already overworked and understaffed nursing department. The palliative care specialists can promote patient self-worth and dignity as past accomplishments are explored, families are brought together to show gratitude, and caring relationships are supported and given a meaningful role to play in the care of their loved one. The palliative care team strives to include family, friends, nursing staff, and anyone in a position to provide physical, spiritual, social, and emotional support to the individual so their needs and expressed hopes are met. The palliative care team knows that hope can be maintained and continues to evolve when a supportive, encouraging, and accepting environment is provided (Duggleby, 2001).

Groopman (2004) wrote about a woman with metastatic breast cancer. The physician had reached a point in her care when no other effective drugs or treatments could be offered. The physician now had the difficult task of informing her. The woman sensed the physician's discomfort and listened to what he had to say. She was saddened by the news and cried briefly but added that now their visits would be her "daily dose of friendship." The patient began to speak of her fears but stopped abruptly when she realized the late hour. She asked the physician if he had the time to listen. The physician had already put in a 10-hour day and knew his family was waiting for him. He regarded their discussion as important as any emergent treatment that required him to stay late. He reached for her hand and reassured her that he had "all the time in the world."

The palliative care team realizes the importance of listening and works with nursing to ensure individuals and their families feel they are being heard, and cared about in this highly technical and impersonal health care environment. A nurse's very presence can instill hope (Ersek & Cotter, 2010).

Persons and families must feel they are more than the disease they are fighting. They must be allowed to keep their dignity and emotional strength intact, so hope can evolve and be redefined as their disease progresses. Nurses can be assisted by the palliative care team to supply the most crucial components necessary for EBh and GBh to evolve. The essential elements so desperately needed by individuals and their families under our care include our presence, our attention, and our empathy. They are truly the greatest gifts we can ever provide.

The foundation of EBh is based in spirituality. An individual's spirituality provides a method to achieve meaning, comfort, and inner peace in his or her life (Groopman, 2004). A patient's spirituality can be expressed through his or her personal methods of coping, religious beliefs, music, art, and what is valued. Enhancing and supporting the patient's spirituality provides a "bridge between hopelessness and meaningfulness in life" (Duggleby, 2001, p. 56). Nurses assisted by the palliative care team can identify and support the spiritual needs of individuals. They can provide a renewed source of hope, and help them to maintain their sense of dignity (Longaker, 1998).

Spirituality plays a very important role in life not just in chronic disease but eventually, in the dying process. It is not solely confined to a patient's faith and religious preference; it is their actual essence. One's spirituality is what makes an individual unique and fosters their sense of hope, defines their suffering, and supports their life journey toward a final sense of peace as they chose to define it. Nurses and the palliative care team must work to identify, support, and promote the individual and his or her family's spiritual needs so they may experience a peaceful resolution and/or acceptance of their personal issues.

The role prayer plays in a patient's life is an important spiritual assessment. Prayer can provide the emotional sense of strength and hope a patient and his or her family may need to meet daily challenges. Prayer can remind us that we are not alone and that we have the love and support of God or a higher spiritual force. The belief in an afterlife and reuniting with loved ones after death provides a source of hope and strength to endure the many hardships during a chronic illness and the dying process. Faith affords the trust that a higher being will remove all pain and suffering. The spiritual beliefs of a loving and merciful God fuel hope and supply a sense of peace and acceptance for many individuals.

The terminally ill and dying and their families can better endure their suffering when they perceive they are spiritually supported. The spiritual counselors and chaplains of the palliative care team can provide this assistance. Prayer or any spiritual ritual requested by the individual or his or her family will bring much needed comfort and assistance. The feelings of support and love these rituals supply are immeasurable, and the effort made to provide them demonstrates respect and a true caring for patients and their families. Faith, religion, and spirituality foster hope.

Individuals and their families need validation of their suffering and emotional pain. They need to trust that others will understand, accept, and respect them, and allow them to safely speak about their feelings (Longaker, 1998). The emotional and physical support provided by nursing and medical staff is essential, and their efforts can be greatly assisted by the palliative care team. Validation of suffering and emotional pain can help to more clearly define and support a patient and family's sense of hope.

> We all need basic human kindness; the reliable presence and love of another person, someone willing to be in regular contact with us for the duration of our journey through suffering. We need others to simply listen and bear witness to our pain, offering support, encouragement, and honesty tempered with compassion. (Longaker, 1998, p. 54)

PHASES OF HOPE

Hope takes on four basic phases for the chronically and terminally ill: hope for a cure, hope for treatment, hope to prolong life, and hope for a peaceful death (Fanslow-Brunjes, 2008). These phases of hope do not necessarily follow in sequence. Individuals and their families can fluctuate back and forth as they attempt to reconcile to each phase. This change and resultant growth process acts more like a pendulum always swinging back and forth until it finds its center and final acceptance. The change and resultant development of hope does not occur from staying in one phase for any given time. It is the continual movement or transitioning through all of the phases of hope that produces the eventual centering. The palliative care team will continue to focus on the individual and family's hopes as they define them, and take on the role of supportive guide. The eventual GBh for a peaceful death can only evolve with the resolution of suffering nurtured by a strong sense of EBh.

Hope for a cure occurs soon after the diagnosis of a chronic and/or terminal illness is made. It is similar to Dr. Kübler-Ross's (1969) stages of grief. The individual and his or her family are in shock, depressed, and in denial. They are angry and are beginning to bargain in an effort to establish some control through prayers and GBh for a cure as they begin to accept what is happening. Health care personnel must be respectful of this phase. It is a highly emotional time. The GBh for a cure requires the acceptance of a terminal disease and introduces the first thoughts of the possibility they may die (Fanslow-Brunjes, 2008). This is a perfect time for the palliative care team to be introduced. A rapport can be established, a needs assessment made, symptom management could be initiated, and spiritual and psychological support would be provided to help strengthen EBh. Focus at this stage is on the GBh for a cure that can only be sustained with a well-supported sense of EBh (Groopman, 2004; Wittenberg-Lyles et al., 2011).

The *hope for treatment* phase develops when the individual learns there are no more options for a cure. Treatments may be available to slow the disease process or provide some additional time (Fanslow-Brunjes, 2008). GBh for a new treatment or acceptance into a new trial study may keep the GBh for a cure alive. Individuals and families at this phase are beginning to build acceptance of the possibility that the disease they are fighting will eventually take their lives. Individuals may cling strongly to one more chemo treatment, or one more surgery that may lead to a possible cure. The palliative care team supports the decision to continue to seek aggressive treatment even in light of a poor prognosis. GBh can be sustained through reinforcement and development of their EBh. Again, EBh is based on the ability to achieve and maintain a sense of dignity, self-worth, and a positive view of the future in the face of hardship, sadness, disease, and misfortune. The palliative care interdisciplinary team's presence will increase with the needs of the individual for symptom management, spiritual, psychological, and emotional support. Any sense of suffering must be controlled so a nurturing environment for EBh can flourish and provide the emotional and spiritual energy to aid in the belief of an individual and his or her family's goals, desires, or wishes (GBh). Hope can be sustained if it is nurtured and suffering is controlled (Scioli & Biller, 2010).

The phase of *hoping to prolong life* can occur at any time during the typically 20- to 40-year chronic and/or terminal illness course. It is most commonly sustained after the hope for a cure has faded (Fanslow-Brunjes, 2008). This phase is marked by the acceptance that a "miracle" may not happen and individuals and families struggle to find some meaning behind their terminal diagnosis. It is in this phase that EBh begins to dominate and there is a gradual shift of focus to comfort care. Transient GBh of wanting to live to see their new grandchildren or to attend the wedding of their daughters may be established. Hope can keep people alive for weeks as they wait for an important event or attempt not to die on someone's birthday or a holiday. Hope keeps individuals alive as they identify the need to instruct family members on financial matters or finalize legal concerns. Time may be needed to prepare families for a life without their loved ones. They become absorbed in the details they feel are important for their loved ones to know. This closure process provides a shift in concentration and can offer a much needed emotional break from their disease process. This type of EBh can impart new energy as emotions are directed to helping their families. It is essential that family members reassure their loved ones that they understand their directions and wishes, and that they will be okay. It is a very difficult conversation to have but the dying often need this reassurance to ease some of the emotional pain the closure process may produce. The bedside nurse and the palliative care team's presence continues to increase in an effort to maintain symptom management, provide emotional and spiritual support, and promote clear communication of individuals' goals of care.

The final phase *hope for a peaceful death* requires intense support of EBh for the individual and family. The GBh for a cure or an additional treatment to obtain more time cannot be sustained without the presence of EBh. The nurse and the palliative care team continue to support the individual and family's hopes as they define them through reinforcement of their emotional and spiritual needs. An individual and family's views of death are unique and must be respected. Many want to fight on with GBh for a miracle, or a new treatment. Issues of futility may not be openly discussed (Fanslow-Brunjes, 2008). Many individuals begin focusing on closure and preparing their family for life without them. It is important to ask what the individual requires for this very emotional time, and to maintain a physical presence to show support and a willingness to assist them in any way possible. Often, the medical team cannot support what they deem futile. The palliative care team recognizes the necessity of including medical staff in the grieving process. There is often a need to explain individual preferences and requests, and emphasize the importance of focusing on sustaining the individual and family's EBh so they can continue to embrace their GBh. It is essential that medical staff refrain from allowing their personal beliefs/ opinions to impact or conflict with the dying individual and the family's specific goals.

> All of us can live with the knowledge that we have an incurable disease, but none of us can live with the thought that we are hopeless. Being labeled hopeless is like being declared a non-being, an object. It is worse than the terminal disease flowing through our body. (Fanslow-Brunjes, 2008, p. 31)

Health care providers must never doubt an individual and his or her family's resilience and capacity to hope. Hope is ever evolving and is a crucial component of living and dying. Hope can transcend suffering and pain on any level whether physical, psychological, spiritual, or emotional. An experienced and dedicated nursing staff and palliative care interdisciplinary team is the key to nurturing and maintaining a patient and family's hopes. Their efforts to support and sustain the GBh and the EBh of individuals under their care is essential. Consulting the palliative care team does not imply physician incompetency, failure, or a lack of trust in the bedside nurse's skills. Rather, it shows an acknowledgment of the necessity for a team approach, and the prioritizing of the physical, emotional, psychological, and spiritual needs of individuals and families so they can continue to hope.

A family's ability to hope is also dependent upon the elimination of their suffering. Their suffering is primarily based on personal stress and anguish over the anticipated death of their loved one. Andershed (2006) noted that families of the dying need to establish feelings of security and trust with their HCPs to successfully manage their grieving and bereavement processes. Authentic and supportive relationships are crucial for good communication and minimizing the stress and associated grieving issues the dying and their families may experience (Bookbinder et al., 2005; Hall, Schroderr, & Weaver, 2002). Without appropriate education and training, HCPs often miss the opportunity to assist a family member and prevent long-term emotional trauma from occurring.

A dying individual's perceived distress can adversely affect immediate and future family stress (Brajtman, 2005; Catlin & Carter, 2002). Long-term psychosocial and mental health issues such as post-traumatic stress disorder (PTSD) can develop as a result of prolonged, unrelieved, stress (Byock, 2012; Ellershaw & Wilkinson, 2011). Negative perceptions of terminal care can influence family coping abilities, grief and bereavement, and future ability to adjust to loss (Brajtman, 2005). There is a continual need for emotional and physical support, reinforcement of decision process, and acknowledgment of the grieving process by nursing and medical staff (Puchalski & Ferrell, 2010).

Any sense of abandonment can be emotionally devastating to an individual in the process of dying and their families (Ferrell & Coyle, 2010; Quill, 1996). Clear and open communication with professional caregiving staff is essential to assist the family in differentiating between suffering and a normal dying process and to comfort the family and assist coping as they witness the death of the loved one (Brajtman, 2005; Catlin & Carter, 2002). Yet, the spiritual and psychosocial needs of the family continue to be ignored, communication is often insufficient or nonexistent, and the assigned nurse is frequently assigned additional duties because of the perceived lack of needs for a dying patient and the family (Becker et al., 2007; Quill, 1996). The absence of this support can result in emotional trauma that will affect a family for the rest of their lives.

The CARES tool was developed to address common deficiencies in knowledge and experience that HCPs encounter when caring for the dying. The CARES tool is not intended to be a replacement for EOL education. It was designed to complement and build upon education obtained from professional organizations such as the Hospice and Palliative Care Nurse Association (HPNA) and the End-of-Life Nursing Education Consortium (ELNEC) project. It is a consolidation of the vast amount of information available on care of the dying into a portable reference that addresses the most common issues a HCP will confront when providing EOL care. It is but one additional resource for nurses and health care professionals to help them promote and sustain hope for the dying and their families.

REFERENCES

Andershed, B. (2006). Relatives in end-of-life care-part I: A systematic review of the literature the last five years, January 1999–February 2004. *Journal of Clinical Nursing, 15*, 1158–1169.

Becker, G., Sarhatlic, R., Olschewski, M., Xander, C., Momm, F., & Blum, H. E. (2007). End-of-life care in hospital: Current practice and potentials for improvement. *Journal of Pain and Symptom Management, 33*(6), 711–719.

Bookbinder, M., Blank, A. E., Arney, E., Wollner, D., Lesage, P., McHugh M., et al. (2005). Improving end of life care: Development and pilot-test of a clinical pathway. *Journal of Pain and Symptom Management, 29*(6), 529–543.

Brajtman, S. (2005). Helping the family through the experience of terminal restlessness. *Journal of Hospice and Palliative Nursing, 7*(2), 73–81.

Byock, I. (1997). *Dying well: Peace and possibilities at the end of life.* New York, NY: Riverhead Books.

Byock, I. (2012). *The best care possible: A physician's quest to transform care through end of life.* New York, NY: Avery.

Catlin, A., & Carter, B. (2002). State of the art. Creation of a neonatal end-of-life palliative care protocol. *Journal of Perinatology, 22*(3), 184–195.

Coward, D. D. (Ed.). (2010). *Pamela G. Reed: Self-transcendence theory* (7th ed.). Maryland Heights, MO: Mosby Elsevier.

Coward, D. D., & Reed, P. G. (1996). Self-transcendence: A resource for healing at the end of life. *Issues in Mental Health Nursing, 17,* 275–288.

Duggleby, W. (2001). Hope at the end of life. *Journal of Hospice and Palliative Care 3*(2), 51–64.

Ellershaw, J., & Wilkinson, S. (2011). *Care of the dying: A pathway to excellence* (2nd ed.). New York, NY: Oxford University Press.

Ersek, M. (Ed.). (2006). *The meaning of hope in the dying* (2nd ed.). New York, NY: Oxford University Press.

Ersek, M., & Cotter, V. T. (2010). The meaning of hope in the dying. In B. Ferrell & N. Coyle (Eds.) *Textbook of palliative care nursing* (3rd ed., pp. 579–595). New York, NY: Oxford University Press.

Fanslow-Brunjes, C. (2008). *Using the power of hope to cope with dying: The four stages of hope.* Sanger, CA: Quill Driver Books/Word Dancer Press.

Ferrell, B. R., & Coyle, N. (Eds.). (2010). *Oxford textbook of palliative nursing* (3rd ed.). New York, NY: Oxford University Press.

Groopman, J. (2004). *Anatomy of hope: How people prevail in the face of illness.* New York, NY: Random House.

Hall, P., Schroderr, C., & Weaver, L. (2002). The last 48 hours of life in long term care: A focused chart audit. *Journal of the American Geriatrics Society, 50*(3), 501–506.

Longaker, C. (1998). *Facing death and finding hope: A guide to the emotional and spiritual care of the dying.* New York, NY: Broadway Books.

Puchalski, C. M., & Ferrell, B. R. (2010). *Making health care whole: Integrating spirituality into patient care.* West Conshohocken, PA: Templeton Press.

Quill, T. E. (1996). *A midwife through the dying process: Stories of healing & hard choices at the end of life.* Baltimore, MA: Johns Hopkins University Press.

Scioli, A., & Biller, H. (2010). *The power of hope.* Deerfield Beach, FL: Health Communications, Inc.

Wicks, R. J. (2012). *Riding the dragon: Ten lessons for inner strength in challenging times.* Notre Dame, IN: Sorin Books.

Wittenberg-Lyles, E., Goldsmith, J., & Ragan, S. (2011). The shift to early palliative care: A typology of illness journeys and the role of nursing. *Clinical Journal of Oncology Nursing, 15*(3), 304–319.

PART VI

Leading Change—Stories and Perspectives From Sunnybrook

CHAPTER 22

Knowledge Translation for Effecting Practice Change

The past decade has seen a notable increase in understanding about the uptake and utilization of scientific evidence in clinical practice and what is necessary to observe improvements in health care. Nevertheless, challenges continue to exist in achieving effective practice change and seeing actual improvements in patient experience and outcomes. Information that can inform practice decision making and lead to improvements in care abounds, but its actual use within daily practice continues to be uneven across practice settings (McCloskey, 2008). A pressing and perplexing issue remains—how to facilitate the appropriate, efficient, and effective transfer of clinically relevant information and technology from discovery and demonstration of its value to routine practice at the point of care with the individual practitioner.

The purpose of this chapter is to highlight what is known about introducing the use of evidence in the daily practice of health care providers and implementing strategies to achieve successful practice change. It is anticipated the information will be useful to those who are leading practice change initiatives in clinical settings.

CONCEPTUALIZING KNOWLEDGE TRANSLATION: UNDERSTANDING THE PROCESS

The ultimate aim of health research in the practice professions is to uncover new knowledge that will aid practitioners in providing safe, effective care and assist them in constantly identifying ways to improve care delivery. To fully accomplish this aim, research must not only be conducted but the knowledge that is uncovered must also be shared so that health care providers and decision

203

FIGURE 22.1 Integrated model for practice improvement.

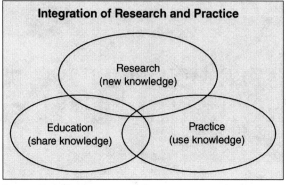

Source: Fitch (1990).

makers have it readily available for their use (Figure 22.1). This implies the need for effective avenues to disseminate any newly discovered knowledge to those who are expected to make use of it and for the implementation of concrete strategies to facilitate the utilization of the knowledge in appropriate ways.

Over the past decade, efforts directed to understanding this process of knowledge translation, which includes knowledge discovery, dissemination, uptake, and utilization (Figure 22.2) has been increasing significantly. There has been a growing realization just how complex the process is and why we need to know more about the various factors that influence whether or not there is a successful outcome. Sharing knowledge and

FIGURE 22.2 Illustration of the key components in the process in knowledge exchange.

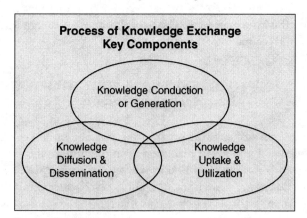

Source: Fitch (2009).

having that knowledge paid attention to, picked up, and actually used in everyday practice is fraught with many potential pitfalls. It is a process that necessitates carefully orchestrated and concerted efforts.

Currently, various conceptualizations exist regarding the process of sharing scientific or research evidence and having it taken up and used in routine clinical practice. The Canadian Institutes of Health Research (CIHR) defines this process of knowledge translation as "the exchange, synthesis, and ethically sound application of research findings within a complex system of relationships among researchers and knowledge users" (CIHR, 2002). A more focused definition for knowledge translation is "the effective and timely incorporation of evidence-based information into the practices of health professionals in such a way so as to effect optimal health care outcomes and maximize the potential for the health system" (University of Toronto, as adapted from the CIHR definition, 2001). Other authors have used terms such as knowledge utilization (Landry, Amara, & Lamari, 2002), knowledge transfer (Eveland, 1986), knowledge mobilization (McCall, Rootman, & Bayley, 2005), knowledge exchange (Lomas, 1993), diffusion of innovations (Rogers, 2003), and knowledge use (Logan & Graham, 1998). Although these terms are often used interchangeably (Grunfeld et al., 2004), each term has a slightly different emphasis on elements of the process that are considered to be of importance.

From the 1960s to the mid-1990s, the process of knowledge translation was seen as primarily a linear one-way process. Knowledge was generated by researchers and seen as a product that could be handed over to the knowledge users through a rather passive process of diffusion (e.g., peer review publications, academic conference presentations). The working assumption was that if the knowledge was made available, the practitioners and policy makers would read it and use it. It was expected the users would embrace the idea of the new knowledge eagerly and be able to use the knowledge easily and appropriately. The process was highly dependent upon the knowledge user seeking out the information and determining what was relevant for his or her practice use.

By the mid-1990s, it was recognized that the knowledge translation process had to use more active dissemination strategies and be two-way; there had to be an exchange between those who generated the knowledge and those who were to use it. The notion of knowledge being embedded and interpreted within a dynamic relationship between the knowledge generators and knowledge users began to emerge as an important element in the process.

It was acknowledged that one needed to understand how new knowledge might need to be adapted for presentation and use within the local practice context if uptake and use of that knowledge was to be successful. Such understanding comes through active, open dialogue, and sharing

FIGURE 22.3 Influences in the knowledge exchange process.

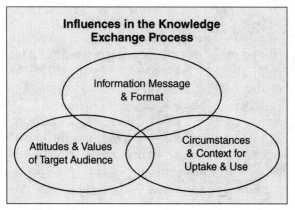

Source: Fitch (2009).

of perspectives from both the evidence and the practice environments. Additionally, the reason it was recognized as a critical factor for success was that the new knowledge or information had to be seen by the knowledge user as being relevant for solving a problem that the user thought was important or of concern. Attention needed to be paid to who the target audience (knowledge user) was expected to be, the type of knowledge that was to be used (i.e., conceptual or technical), how it was expected to be used, the format for the presentation of the information (i.e., words, graphic, pictures, protocols, pathway documents, etc.), and the users' attitudes about both the problem and the proposed solution using the new information (Figure 22.3). If the new information was not seen by the users as relevant for solving the problem they had identified, or if using it was seen as creating hassles, more difficulties, or taking unnecessary time in their already busy day, they would not move to embrace and utilize it. The knowledge could easily be set aside and ignored (Blasi, Harkness, Ernst, Georgiou, & Kleijnen, 2001; Grol & Grimshaw, 2003). Having a clear description of how the knowledge or innovation was expected to be taken up and used was necessary to reduce uncertainty. This description needed to include details about what will change as a result of using the knowledge, where the changes will be observed, and what impacts will be felt by whom.

Since 2000, there has been an added realization that having new knowledge or information and having tools that summarize that knowledge (i.e., guidelines, standards, pathways, protocols, etc.) is simply not enough to achieve lasting practice change (Grol & Grimshaw, 2003). There is a need for a far more active and intentional approach to introducing new evidence in a practice setting. In particular, social strategies and working partnerships are key elements for successful uptake and utilization of knowledge in daily practice. Practice behavior change occurs through people and relationships, shared agendas, and mutual agreement about what needs to be accomplished. The organizational context, the attitudes and existing knowledge held by the target audience members (knowledge users), the expected impact on practice behaviors of using the new information, the capacity of the users to actually utilize the information, and the active support of champions and agency leaders were recognized as vitally important aspects of successful implementation (Montague, 2006). Without attention to the full range of influencing factors, little success could be expected in having practitioners make use of the new knowledge in their daily practice.

The most significant development regarding knowledge translation during recent years has been the shift from focusing on the perspective of the individual practitioner to understanding the influence of the wider system in which the practitioner works. Clearly the process of knowledge translation is complex (Larsen, 1980); interactive (Rogers, 2002); and reliant on the user's knowledge, beliefs, and experiences (National Centre for the Dissemination of Disability Research, 1996). Multiple factors come into play in any one situation to effect practice behavior change. But if implementation is to be successful and practice behavior change sustained, attention must be given to the system level perspective as well. The context or environment in which a practitioner or an inter-professional team works and provides care contains influences that can foster or hinder a successful outcome. Union approaches, management policies, professional regulations, institutional priorities, and available resources are examples of potential influences. Making use of new knowledge and achieving sustained practice change may require the acquisition of new resources, significant education and capacity building, different facilities, and enhanced staff support.

Systems model thinking brings forward the notion of knowledge integration for sustained practice change (Best, 2006). Any implementation of new knowledge will be introduced into a setting that has existing priorities, culture, and context; knowledge uptake will be mediated through relationships (likely multiple) within the organization throughout the implementation cycle; and the degree of its use over time will be a function of how embedded it can become within practitioner behaviors, and institutional programs and policy mandates. Is use of the new information clearly stated in job descriptions? Is performance regarding its use incorporated into performance reviews? Are there clearly stated expectations for documenting practice with the new knowledge? Does use of the new knowledge become a new standard of care or practice policy? Are there observable repercussions if the new practice is not followed?

The planning of the implementation cycle for use of new information ought to take into account how the several levels in the organization will make use of the new information or innovation—the individual practitioner, the group or team, and the system or policy level. What it actually means to "use" the new information should be clearly articulated. For example, implementing the use of a new screening tool for psychosocial distress may allow the following:

▨ The practitioner reviews the data from the patient during a clinic appointment and uses it to open a discussion with the individual and cocreate a plan of action with the person to manage fatigue.

▨ The interprofessional team reviews the data at team meetings to determine what patient issues need to be a priority for them to develop team responsibilities concerning fatigue.

▨ The educator reviews the data to identify what educational programs or resources are required for patients or for health care professionals.

▨ The manager evaluates documentation about fatigue by staff members to provide feedback during performance appraisals.

▨ The operational director cites the data about fatigue to advocate for more resources to design a fatigue clinic.

▨ The executive director quotes the information about fatigue to signify organizational priorities for person-centered care.

Action-oriented implementation strategies are necessary at all levels in an organization to achieve success in knowledge translation and integration. Sustained practice change requires multiple approaches or implementation strategies. However, the specific implementation strategies that will be successful at one level will not necessarily be effective on another. Approaches need to be designed for each of the levels within an organization. Greenhalgh, Robert, MacFarlane, Bate, and Kyriakidou (2004) have written extensively about what factors need to be considered by the individuals who are leading an implementation effort. Focused planning is needed at all three levels when trying to achieve effective and sustained knowledge translation outcomes.

For example, influencing practice change on the part of individual practitioners has a great deal to do with individual personality traits, perceptions, and coping styles; influencing practice change at a team or organizational level is more about social networks and relationships, opinion leaders, incentives, and team skills; influencing systems or policy change is about use of credible champions, boundary spanners, formal programs, and an organization's capacity for change and innovation (Greenhalgh et al., 2004).

At all organizational levels, the new knowledge or evidence needs to be seen as credible and required for necessary improvement, and the message inherent in the evidence needs to be relevant to the members of the target audience (i.e., help them solve a problem they are experiencing). Political will and personal agendas on the part of leaders within the organization can facilitate and foster an implementation plan or can thwart and destroy the effort. Clearly this aspect needs to be assessed carefully prior to any launch of an initiative. Strategies will be needed to influence the political will and ensure there is organizational support for the implementation.

Finally, successful implementation will require a thoughtful and detailed social strategy to inform all stakeholders and engage those expected to utilize any new knowledge or innovation. Communication about what will be gained by using the new knowledge and how it is to be used should be shared early in the implementation and repeated regularly. Throughout the various stages of the implementation, regular updates about progress and feedback about what is being accomplished help to generate energy for continuing to engage in the initiative.

Engaging the members of the intended audience—the individuals who are expected to "use" the new knowledge or information—throughout the implementation planning and activity is critical for success. There are many ways this can be accomplished: focus groups, surveys, team meetings, task group membership, and seeking feedback (on paper or electronically). Their views on all aspects of the implementation will be useful for identifying potential barriers to implementation, facilitators to use of the new knowledge, and what success could actually look like. Knowledge users need to be true partners in the process.

PLANNING FOR KNOWLEDGE IMPLEMENTATION

Given that the process of knowledge implementation is so complex, planning an effective introduction of a new innovation or practice must be done carefully and with intention. Successful planning ought to incorporate guidance from models of change management, diffusion of innovation theory, principles of adult learning, and learning from social marketing (Fitch, 2009).

One predominant model that can be helpful in planning for the introduction and development of the implementation strategy for a new clinical practice change was designed by Graham and colleagues (2006) (Figure 22.4). This model emphasizes (see center of Figure 22.4) the need to have the new knowledge uncovered through research and literature, synthesized into a clear statement about the implications for practice, and formatted into a distinct knowledge product or tool (i.e., review paper, clinical guideline, protocol, pathway, etc). The decision about what format the knowledge product or tool should take ought to reflect its intended use and dissemination strategy. For example, raising awareness may be achieved with a review paper in an academic audience or may be more effectively achieved through the use of a case study video or theatrical presentation in a clinical audience. Advancing knowledge or skill may require instructional modules and practice guides. Changing practice behavior may be supported

FIGURE 22.4 Model used to guide planning for the knowledge transfer process.

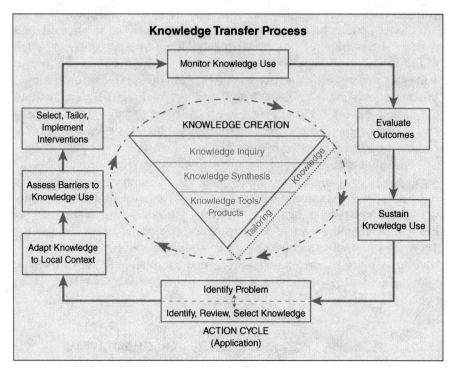

Source: Graham, Logan, Harrison, et al. (2006).

most effectively through collaboratively designing procedural protocols and clinical guidelines or pathways together as an interprofessional team.

The identified implication for practice change becomes the key message for the knowledge translation process. It is the foundation for communication and clearly defining expectations of the practitioner or knowledge user in making actual use of the knowledge or information. Being clear about what is expected of the practitioner in using the new knowledge or a new innovation is important for success. If there is uncertainty about how to utilize the new information and what is expected in terms of practitioner behavior, the practitioner will feel discomfort and heightened distress in trying to perform appropriately.

The implementation steps of the knowledge translation process demand clear engagement with the members (expected knowledge users) of the local clinical setting to determine the nature of the clinical problem that can be solved with the new information, what the reality of the local situation is for using the information (i.e., barriers, challenges,

facilitators, etc.), and what actual format needs to be used to disseminate the knowledge and support its uptake and utilization in the clinical setting.

The effectiveness of various dissemination strategies is highlighted in
Table 22.1. It is important to select dissemination strategies that are effective
for the specific goals or objectives of the knowledge translation initiative.
For example, if the intention is one of raising awareness about the need
for change, this would require different strategies than actually changing
attitudes or improving practice skills to be effective. Early and ongoing
engagement with potential knowledge users is a critical aspect in planning for the implementation of new knowledge use and selecting the most
effective approaches for the local setting and target audience. What might be

TABLE 22.1
Strategies to Achieve Specific Knowledge Translation Objectives

Pathman-PRECEED Model for Knowledge Translation Perspective of Target (Policy Maker, Consumer, or Clinician)				
INTERVENTION	RAISE AWARENESS	OBTAIN AGREEMENT	ENCOURAGE ADOPTION	SUPPORT ADHERENCE
Predisposing	Distribution of printed information; journals; media campaigns; lectures; rounds; academic detailing			
Enabling		Opinion leaders; small group sessions for clinicians	Small group sessions for clinicians; patient education methods; clinical flowcharts or algorithms; academic detailing	
Reinforcing			Small group sessions for audit and feedback	Reminders (professional and patient), multiple interventions

Source: Davis, Evans, Jadad, et al. (2003).

effective with one group of users (i.e., palliative care nurses, operating room nurses, social workers) may not be as effective with others (i.e., surgeons, palliative care physicians, pharmacists). Table 22.2 highlights strategies that will achieve changes in knowledge, skill, or practice change. It is important to select the strategies that are effective in achieving the desired result of an initiative.

PRINCIPLES FOR IMPLEMENTING KNOWLEDGE TRANSLATION

The following principles for implementing a knowledge translation initiative were devised following an extensive review of relevant literature related to knowledge translation and experience working across Canada implementing several innovations in practice (Fitch, Nicoll, & Bennie, 2012). The principles capture aspects that ought to be taken into consideration when developing a plan to launch an innovation that aims to change practice in health care.

TABLE 22.2
Effectiveness of Various Implementation
Strategies for Specific Outcomes

EFFECTIVENESS OF IMPLEMENTATION STRATEGIES IN ACHIEVING SPECIFIC GOALS	How effective are strategies?		
	IMPROVE KNOWLEDGE AND ATTITUDES	IMPROVE SKILLS	CHANGE PRACTICE
Educational outreach visits	+	?	+
Workshops with interactions	+	+	+
Reminders	+	?	+
Social marketing	+	?	+
Multifaceted approaches	+	?	+
Opinion leaders	+	?	+/=
Patient mediated strategies	?	–	+/=
Audit & feedback	+	?	+/=
Educational materials	+	?	–
Didactic conferences	+	–	–
Local consensus processes	+	?	–

Sources: Cheater et al. (2009); Grimshaw, Eccles, Lavis, Hill, and Squires (2012).

1. **Problem assessment/understanding**

   a. Definition: Early identification of a problem or issue, supported by evidence, and the subsequent introduction of appropriate knowledge to address the problem or issue of concern

   b. Action: Begin with a careful assessment of the nature of the problem that has been identified; understand the issue from the perspective of all stakeholders; and use a variety of methods to capture the perspectives

2. **Tailoring to local context**

   a. Definition: Adapting an innovation to suit the local situation, organization characteristics, patient needs, and available resources

   b. Action: Seek to understand the local environment and setting; what is the capacity to implement the use of the new knowledge or innovation; what adaptations will be necessary to fit the local culture and ways of working

3. **Assessment of individual perceptions/motivation**

   a. Definition: Examination of individual values, beliefs, credibility of the knowledge, behaviors toward sustaining the knowledge, beliefs about capabilities, confidence, and emotional response to the knowledge

   b. Action: Seek to understand what interpretations are being given to the problem and to the anticipated solution by all stakeholders; identify the various motivations that are driving participants' involvement in the initiative

4. **Barrier identification/management**

   a. Definition: Assessment of the local situation for barriers that may impede or limit uptake of knowledge and devise targeted interventions to minimize or remove them

   b. Action: Identify the potential for barriers that will block or slow the uptake and utilization of the new approach; barriers may be on the part of people or on the part of the environmental capacity; preparations for change and capacity to cope with change are to be assessed; identify potential facilitators that will support the initiative to move forward

5. **Identification of social influences**

   a. Definition: Recognize and promote positive role models, opinion leaders, and social supports and address negative social influences

b. Action: Identification of individuals within the environment who are role models or have leadership characteristics/capacity (who can influence others); it is key to have senior leadership individuals involved

6. **Training and/or coaching**

a. Definition: Enhancing understanding of new knowledge and developing skills for implementing that knowledge

b. Action: Consider what education and training (skill development) will be required to actually use the new information in practice

7. **Organizational capacity building/infrastructure development**

a. Definition: Organizations must be ready for change and exhibit a cultural fit with the innovation; infrastructure must dedicate human and financial resources

b. Action: Identify the strengths/weaknesses within the organization to support any change that is necessary; what resources can be leveraged or will need to be added (people, materials, expertise)

8. **Patient engagement and implementation**

a. Definition: With any innovation, patients and families must be informed of it, be aware of its scope, understand their role in it, and be able to participate in its implementation and evaluation

b. Action: Devise methods to engage patients and family members in the efforts early and continuously; utilize their input as advice for the work

9. **Monitoring, evaluation, and reporting**

a. Definition: Setting of specific and measurable aims for an innovation and process of continuous quality improvement

b. Action: Devise ways of monitoring progress and evaluating success; make use of quantitative and qualitative data: report the results and share stories regularly with all stakeholders

10. **Dissemination**

a. Definition: Results and lessons learned from an innovation must be shared with relevant stakeholders/audiences (internal and external)

b. Action: Share descriptions of progress and success throughout the implementation cycle; share a description of what worked and what did not work with external colleagues in the field

In summary, success in achieving actual practice change is challenging and takes intentional strategy design (Howell, Hack, Green, & Fitch, 2014). Effective implementation and sustained outcomes are more likely to occur when the following axioms are incorporated into the planning:

1. Single behavior change is set out clearly; innovation itself is clearly described
2. Members of the target group are involved early and throughout the project
3. Active strategies are used to educate intended users
4. Multiple channels are used to communicate throughout the project
5. Focus on influencing multiple audiences, each with a specific goal
6. Use of credible sources for knowledge and opinion leaders
7. Modification of systems as required for use of the innovation
8. Clearly established links between developers and end-users
9. Clearly stated benefits and demands of the innovation when it is in use

KEY CONSIDERATIONS FOR IMPLEMENTING KNOWLEDGE TRANSLATION: SUPPORTING PEOPLE AND MANAGING CHANGE

Introduction of a new practice innovation will necessitate working with individuals, all of whom will have what is called a "mindset," or a way of thinking about and seeing the world around them and how it works. Whether or not a new innovation is seen as contrary to their views has a significant influence on how they perceive and respond to that innovation. In the words of Bagehot in 1873 (cited in Rogers):

> One of the greatest pains to human nature is the pain of a new idea. It . . . makes you think that after all, your favorite notions may be wrong, your firmest beliefs may be ill-founded . . . naturally, therefore, common men hate a new idea, and are disposed more or less to ill-treat the original man who brings it.

The attitudes and values of individuals will color or influence the perception of an innovation message or anticipated change in practice. Often, health care professionals see the expectation of using new knowledge as an implied criticism that they have not been doing a good job, despite the reality the knowledge was not previously available to them. Work by Gabbay and le May (2004) reinforced Bagehot's view as they identified that "clinicians rarely accessed, appraised, and used explicit evidence directly from research . . . instead they replied on 'mind-lines,' collectively reinforced, internalized, tacit guidelines" (p. 1015). Breaking through these "mind-lines" is a considerable challenge, especially in the acute care settings of today, which can be described as ones of escalating patient caseloads, increasing complexity of treatment protocols, and decreasing financial resources.

Rogers (2003) describes individuals falling in several major categories related to their openness to and engagement with change. The innovators and early adopters are ahead of the rest, risk-takers who are ready to try something new. The majority of individuals in an organization can be categorized into either early or late adopters in picking up and utilizing the innovation. The last group contains the laggards, who are the least open to change and the last to engage in adopting new innovations and embracing change. Strategies to engage and support each of these groups will need to be different. In general, human beings experience heightened anxiety with changes in their environment and habits and it takes time to adjust and find a "new normal." Support during these times of uncertainty and adjustment is an important consideration for successful outcomes.

The nature of change also makes demands upon individuals. Change may be conceptualized as developmental, transitional, or transformational. Developmental change is focused on improvement of what currently exists within defined parameters. Transitional change is a replacement of the existing state with a new state. The common characteristics of these types of changes include:

- Outcomes can be quantified and known in advance of implementation
- Significant culture, behavior, or mindset change is not required
- The change process, its resource requirements, and timetable (for the most part) can be managed

However, transformational change is radical change from one state to another. Its characteristics are:

- The future state cannot be completely known in advance
- Significant transformations of the organization's culture and people's behavior and mindsets are required
- The change process itself cannot be tightly managed or controlled (future is unknown and human dynamics too unpredictable)

Transformational change is the most challenging type of change to cope with for all concerned and demands different types of messaging and support throughout the process than with developmental or transitional change. It is important to identify whether the introduction of new knowledge and an innovation is going to require developmental, transitional, or transformational change. The last, of course, has the largest magnitude and impact on staff as well as potential for significant practice change.

SUGGESTED STEPS FOR SPECIFIC PLANNING

The following list of topics highlights steps for action and areas to be considered in planning a knowledge translation initiative within a clinical setting.

A. Understand the current/existing reality of the setting (Assessment at the onset as a basis for planning using various methods—quantitative and qualitative)

- Environment/context for change
- Readiness for change/capacity to engage in change/how adaptive is the organization
  - Shared goals
  - Responsibility for success
  - Collegiality
  - Continuous improvement
  - Lifelong learning
  - Risk taking
  - Supportive and inclusive
  - Mutual respect
  - Openness/discussion and questions welcomed
  - Change and challenge seen as an opportunity
  - Innovation and creativity seen as values
  - Celebration and humor
- Barriers to change/threats
  - Environment
    - Structural (decision making, physical, incentives)
    - Social (politics, personalities, local champions, culture and beliefs)
    - Patients
    - Medical–legal
  - Individual
    - Knowledge/beliefs
    - Motivation/attitudes
    - Values/behavior
    - Skills/perceptions
    - Socialization of health care provider
    - View of innovation (compatible, relative advantage, complexity, observability, trialability)
- Culture of the setting
- Support of leadership for change
- Strengths and opportunities

B. Determine what needs to change to see improvements in which areas
- Set out a vision (shared with all stakeholders)
- Aims (be specific about desired and intended outcomes)

▓ Goals (be specific about what is to be achieved)
▓ Desired results (be specific about what will constitute success)

C. Design an intervention or implementation strategy

▓ Identify what actions are needed to create the practice change you want to achieve
▓ Tailor interventions for setting, barriers identified, target audience, and stage of implementation
▓ Determine who (individual/organization) can be a partner in the implementation
▓ Identify any opportunities for integration with existing initiatives

D. Think strategically/plan intentionally

▓ What to do to "unfreeze" the current situation
▓ What to do to hold on through the change and live through it
▓ How to embed the "new" in the actual practice behavior
▓ Set out evaluation:
  • Intervention happening/outcome achieved/accountability mechanism
▓ Work the interplay of evidence, context, and facilitation (defined strategies)

E. Design a specific action plan

▓ Roles and responsibilities (who will do what)—individuals and groups; do they have the necessary knowledge and skill to manage the project
▓ Target audience(s) for action
▓ Activities according to timelines (approach—launch and follow-up, phase over time, staged by group or setting, multi-pronged, etc.)
▓ Communication strategy (messages, to whom, frequency, format)
▓ Milestones (deliverables)
▓ Evaluation metrics (monitor progress, hold all accountable, see where to improve)
▓ Facilitative strategies for staff engagement (input, problem solving, decision making)
  • Dedicated time for staff (i.e., unit champions, councils, mentors)
  • Clear expectations (frequently stated)
  • Regular use of appreciative inquiry approaches, encouraging dialogue and questioning
  • Provision of incentives ("the right ones"; recognition and reward)
  • Provide (personal, relevant) metrics
  • Time for learning and adjustment
  • Rapid cycle orientation ("just try it")
  • What resources need to be added

F. Determine sustainability for new practice

▓ Embed innovation in organizational memory
▓ Incorporate new practice into the routine workflow

- Set out documentation requirements
- Insert expectations for performance into roles and responsibilities
- Build requirements into policies/procedures
- Link to/build on/integrate with existing (successful) initiatives
- Incorporate relevant learning into educational events
- Where possible, build capacity for structural, social, and human resource capital for "new practice"

SUMMARY

Evidence-based care offers the means to improve and refine practice to ensure optimal outcomes, but concerted effort is needed for effective diffusion, dissemination, uptake, utilization, and integration of relevant evidence. Not only must practitioners at the point of care actively engage in the knowledge translation process, but organizations need to ensure the environment is supportive of the necessary change that will come about as evidence is used to change patient experience with health care.

REFERENCES

Best, A. (2006, February). *Integrating knowledge strategies: New models for more effective action*. Paper presented at the OBCCRI Workshop on Knowledge Exchange, Toronto, ON, Canada.

Blasi, Z. D., Harkness, E., Ernst, E., Georgious, A., & Kleijnen, J. (2001). Influence of context effects on health outcomes: A systematic review. *Lancet, 357,* 757–762.

Canadian Institutes of Health Research. (2002). Knowledge translation fact sheet. Retrieved from www.cihr-irsc.gc.ca/e26574.html

Cheater, F., Baker, R., Gillies, C., Hearnshaw, H., Flottorp, S., Robertson, N., & Oxman, A. D. (2009). Tailored interventions to overcome identified barriers to change: Effects on professional practice and health care outcomes. *Cochrane Database of Systematic Reviews, 4.*

Eveland, J. D. (1986). Diffusion, technology transfer and implementation. *Knowledge, 8,* 303–322.

Fitch, M. I. (2009). Moving knowledge: The possibilities and complexities of qualitative and participatory research. In J. J. Nelson, J. Gould, & S. Keller-Olaman (Eds.), *Cancer on the margins: Method and meaning in participatory research* (chapter 12, pp. 252–268). Toronto, ON: University of Toronto Press.

Fitch, M. I., Nicoll, I., & Bennie, F. (2012, August). *Achieving person-centered care: The need for multiple strategies*. Poster presented at the International Union against Cancer Congress, Montreal, QC, Canada.

Gabbay, J., & le May, A. (2004). Evidence-based guidelines or collectively constructed "mindlines"? Ethnographic study of knowledge management in primary care. *British Medical Journal, 329,* 1013–1017.

Graham, I. D., Logan, J., Harrison, M. B., Straus, S. E., Tetroe, J., Caswell, W., & Robinson, N. (2006). Lost in knowledge translation: Time for a map. *Journal of Continuing Education in the Health Professions, 26*, 13–24.

Greenhalgh, T., Robert, G., MacFarlane, F., Bate, P., & Kyriakidou, O. (2004). Diffusion of innovations in service organizations: Systematic review and recommendations. *Milbank eQuarterly, 82*, 581–629.

Grimshaw, J. M., Eccles, M. P., Lavis, J. N., Hill, S. J., & Squires, J. E. (2012). Knowledge translation of research findings. *Implementation Science, 7*, 50.

Grol, R., & Grimshaw, J. (2003). From best evidence to best practice: Effective implementation of change in patient care. *Lancet, 362*, 1225–1230.

Grunfeld, E., Zitzelsberger, L., Hayter, C., Berman, N., Cameron, R., Evans, W. K., & Stern, H. (2004). The role of knowledge translation for cancer control in Canada. *Chronic Diseases in Canada, 25*(2), 1–6.

Howell, D., Hack, T. F., Green, E., & Fitch, M. (2014). Cancer distress screening data: Translating knowledge into clinical action for quality response. *Palliative and Supportive Care, 12*, 39–51.

Landry, R., Amara, N., & Lamari, M. (2002). Climbing the ladder of research utilization: Evidence from social research. *Science Communication, 22*, 396–422.

Larsen, J. K. (1980). Knowledge utilization: What it is? *Knowledge: Creation, Diffusion, Utilization, 1*, 421–443.

Logan, J., & Graham, I. D. (1998). Toward a comprehensive interdisciplinary model of health care research use. *Science Communication, 20*, 227–246.

Lomas, J. (1993). Diffusion, dissemination, and implementation: Who should do what? *Annals of New York Academy of Science, 703*, 226–235.

McCall, D. S., Rootman, I. & Bayley, D. (2005). International School Health Network: An informal network for advocacy and knowledge exchange. *Promotional Health, 12*(3), 173–177.

McCloskey, D. J. (2008). Nurses' perceptions of research utilization in a corporate health care system. *Journal of Nursing Scholarship, 40*, 39–45.

Montague, T. (2006). Patient-provider partnerships in health care: Enhancing knowledge translation and improving outcomes. *Healthcare Papers, 7*(2), 56–61.

National Centre for the Dissemination of Disability Research. (1996). A review of the literature on dissemination and knowledge utilization. NCDDR. Retrieved from www.ncddr.org/du/products/review/index.html

Rogers, E. M. (2002). The nature of technology transfer. *Science Communication, 23*, 323–341.

Rogers, E. M. (2003). *Diffusion of innovation* (5th ed.). New York, NY: Free Press.

University of Toronto. (2001). As adapted from the CIHR definition. Definition available at http://www.ktp.utoronto.ca/whatisktp/definition

CHAPTER 23

Leading Change—Stories and Perspectives

You will quickly see that this chapter takes a very different approach. You have now spent time thinking about the current literature and evidence related to improving care at the end of life (EOL) through caring and compassion. You have read that there is an imperative to improve the way we interact, relate, and care for those who are dying and their families. You have seen how the CARES tool can be effectively used in clinical practice to improve both life and death, just as it did with our case study of Steven. You have also reviewed organizational change models that provide frameworks for translating this knowledge into action. But, where do we go from here? What is our role as care providers and leaders to facilitate the effective transfer of this evidence into clinical practice? What is our role in influencing those around us to collectively integrate the evidence more broadly? What is our role to lead practice change and innovation by designing structures and processes to not only integrate the evidence, but to support staff to do so and to sustain those changes over time?

Together let's explore how we might use the earlier evidence to influence your thinking, change behavior, and clinical practice across an organization, and set us on a path to change lives. This chapter is a story of shared narratives. I use stories from my own life, the lives of those around me, strangers who I have met along the way, families who have lost loved ones, and health care providers. I share with you one organization's experience and journey in moving knowledge to action, through the corporate implementation of the "Comfort Measures Strategy," which fully integrates the CARES tool.

I describe the application of this tool at Sunnybrook Health Sciences Centre through our story of how we developed a vision for quality dying, engaged a passionate team, and began our first steps through the development, implementation, and evaluation of our Comfort Measures Strategy. This includes describing how the CARES tool is currently being used, including the supporting tools and resources, the roles of the interprofessional team members, education and professional development to build capacity, and ongoing evaluation. I also describe the infrastructure we have built to support knowledge translation for best practice implementation, and the foundation of person-centered care, upon which it is built. I hope that by sharing an example of how knowledge can be moved to action, our experience may assist you in your future endeavors to support the broader application of this model into clinical practice.

WHY STORIES AND NARRATIVES?

Knowledge translation and change management theory was previously discussed in great detail, highlighting how the CARES tool, as an evidence-based framework, can support our vision of practice change. As we all know, implementing change is complex. When we talk about moving evidence to practice, what are we hoping will happen? Attention must be paid to implementing and evaluating interventions that change behavior to reflect current evidence. This process by which knowledge translates into actionable behavior has been viewed as the "black box phenomenon" (Estabrooks, Wallin, & Milner, 2003), recognizing that there are many mediating factors that influence knowledge uptake, including those such as education, experience, organizational context, and administrative support.

And then, in a very different moment, as I sat at my daughter's dance class reading the book *The Last Lecture*, an insight came to me about the use and impact of stories. *The Last Lecture* is a book that was written by a computer science professor named Randy Pausch (Pausch & Zaslow, 2008), who was asked to give a "last lecture," a common practice for professors to impart their deepest insights. Because Pausch had been diagnosed with terminal cancer, the lecture, in fact, became his last lecture, where he shared his wisdom for life. In the Foreword of this book, written by his wife Jai, she shared how amazed she is at how Randy has inspired so many. She notes that his book has been used in classrooms and has been assigned reading. She has received countless letters from those students who talk about how his words have changed their lives.

In another well-known book, the *New York Times* bestseller *Kitchen Table Wisdom: Stories That Heal*, Rachel Naomi Remen (2006) shares her idea that stories have the power to heal. In the Foreword of this book, we learn that stories are the language of community, and there is a great hunger for a feeling of connection. Stories inspire the heart and connect us to each other in meaningful ways, providing the opportunity to open the door to transformation. "We all have within us access to a greater wisdom, and we may not even know that until we speak out loud" (Remen, 2006).

I felt compelled to ask myself why these books inspired me. What was it about the words, the stories, the heart strings they pulled at that spoke to me, and caused me to *want* to share these stories? Why did I share the YouTube link for Randy's lecture thinking that these stories might also resonate with others? And they did. I found myself wondering if we could create the same energy for EOL care at our institution and beyond.

If we return to the literature, we learn that in the narrative tradition, the diffusion of innovations within organizations gives a shared story, and interventions can be directed toward supporting "communities of practice" with a positive story to tell (Bate, 2004). If we embrace the important dimension of organizational innovativeness, an innovative organization is one in which stories can be told and there is the capacity to capture and circulate these stories. Storytelling clarifies one's thinking and describes a context and event within that context, including observable patterns and connections (Zimmerman, Lindberg, & Plsek, 1998). Might we be able to create a story about how an organization changed the perspective of "quality dying"? Might we be able to change the way a nation tells the story of quality dying?

OUR QUALITY DYING STORY BEGINS

To provide some context, I begin by describing Sunnybrook Health Sciences Centre (Sunnybrook) as an organization. This is important because it helps set the stage for the vastness of our goal to integrate the CARES tool into daily clinical care. Additionally, I provide an overview of Sunnybrook's corporate quality dying initiative (QDI) that has provided the structure, support, and oversight for the accomplishments to date. Sunnybrook is one of Canada's largest academic health science centers and is fully affiliated with the University of Toronto. Sunnybrook's mandate is to care for patients and their families when "it matters most." The vision is to invent the future of health care, based on the values of excellence, collaboration, accountability, respect, and engagement. It began as a hospital for Canadian veterans and has flourished into a fully affiliated teaching hospital of the University of Toronto, evolving to meet the needs of a diverse growing community. Sunnybrook is program based, with eight programs across three campuses. Sunnybrook provides care for 1.2 million patient visits each year, has more than 10,000 staff and 2,000 volunteers, and teaches, more than 4,000 students each year.

As a quaternary academic health sciences center with internationally recognized cancer and trauma programs, death and dying are significant elements of our institution's overall patient and family care experience. Based on 2008–2009 and 2009–2010 data (fiscal), in our acute care setting there was an average of 29,918 admissions and 922 (3.1%) deaths occurring each year, equating to approximately 18 deaths per week. It was noted that the majority of these deaths occurred in the acute care setting. We began to realize that there were opportunities to improve the physical, emotional, and practical needs of dying patients and their families.

A SHARED VISION FOR QUALITY DYING

It is well known that effectively diagnosing dying is a complex process influenced by many factors. Adding to this, clinicians in general receive limited training regarding knowledge and skills related to both diagnosing dying and the care elements comprising excellent EOL care. Factoring in the general societal perceptions and expectations regarding the ability to cure disease/illness, we were aware that our clinicians were challenged to consistently provide quality care for our dying patients. Some of these challenges were related to system issues and some had been associated with practices such as advance care planning, clarifying goals of care, making decisions for escalation of care related to patient and family preferences, and overall provision of symptom management at the EOL. However, our primary impetus for the development of the QDI was David's story. David had been transferred from the critical care unit to a ward where he was to be given comfort care. We are very sad to say, this was not his experience. David passed away the next afternoon. At the end of his life, he experienced significant pain and shortness of breath. David's daughter, Susan, advocated for her father, by sharing their story on video with Sunnybrook and challenging us to rethink EOL care and change the care of future patients. The result was the development of the QDI and we began our journey to transform care of the dying.

The vision of the QDI is that *dying patients and the families receive the highest quality of care*, regardless of the setting of care. This means that all patients receive the same quality of care whether they die in a setting where EOL care is a primary focus, such as the palliative care unit, or whether they die in an acute care or medical/surgical clinical setting. The corporate QDI Steering Committee was created to set the direction for the work that was to unfold. This committee is an interprofessional team of individuals who are passionate about quality dying and represent clinical programs and settings across the organization. The team also includes integral departmental partners including the palliative care consult team (PCCT), quality and patient safety, spiritual care, and ethics. This team of dedicated individuals initially set the stage by completing a number of significant activities essential to assessing need, exploring organizational context and perspectives of stakeholders, and determining the specific intervention to be implemented.

PLANNING FOR KNOWLEDGE IMPLEMENTATION

Our work was divided into two phases, with the first phase primarily exploring the current challenges and potential opportunities, to inform what would become our first specific intervention. There were several key areas of activity and I describe each of those in more detail. At the foundation of all our discussion was the commitment to ensure that our strategy was person centered and informed by those for whom we care.

As a beginning step, we completed an extensive review of the literature to explore the care elements that families perceived as most important to their care at the EOL. The synthesis identified eight core domains:

1. Pain and symptom management
2. Timely and clear communication
3. Information to prepare families for approaching death
4. Spirituality/dignity/respect
5. Person-centered decision making
6. Practical needs of the family
7. Supportive needs of the family
8. Caregiver satisfaction with hospital facilities/staff

This analysis was extremely important to our team, as it provided us with the opportunity to see through the eyes of patients and families. As each concept was reviewed, the experience of the patient and family was brought front and center. Our priority was to ensure that the strategy would provide care and caring that was personal and compassionate, while supporting the complex multidimensional needs of patients and families in the most meaningful way. We also found it was interesting to learn that the identified domains aligned very closely with the domains of our corporate Patient Experience Survey, issued through the National Research Corporation of Canada (NRCC). As a health care organization in Ontario, we are legislated through the Excellent Care for All Act (ECFAA), which came into law in June 2010, to be accountable for the delivery of high-quality care, including the requirement to have patient surveys in place to evaluate care. What was even more important to learn was that our current survey did not provide the opportunity to receive feedback on EOL care. This was identified as a gap and highlighted the need to develop and implement a new survey focused on EOL care.

As a result, a second literature review was completed to explore survey implementation to evaluate the family experience of EOL. Predeveloped surveys were evaluated for their ability to measure the family experience within the domains we had identified from the literature. Two surveys were identified that best aligned with the domains. The first was the CANHELP (Canadian Health Care Evaluation Project) questionnaire, which was designed to evaluate satisfaction with care for older patients with life-threatening illnesses and their family members. The second tool we reviewed was an EOL tool available through NRCC, which had been developed by Casey House, a specialized organization providing care and community outreach programs for individuals with HIV. Following a careful review of each tool, including the content and purpose of each question, we felt that we needed to create a new questionnaire. Our product was the NRCC EOL Family Satisfaction Questionnaire.

With our newfound learning about the areas of care that are most important to persons and families and a new tool that would potentially provide us with the opportunity to seek ongoing feedback from families about the care we provided, we had a starting point for "something." However, the big questions were, "What were we going to implement?" and "How did we know that we were truly going to design a strategy that would make a difference from the perspective of those for whom we cared?" In keeping with our commitment to patients and families, we knew family engagement was our priority. So we began a process to invite families that had lost a loved one at Sunnybrook to share their stories and tell us about their experiences. As a team, we were keenly aware that great thought, sensitivity, and planning were required to make this happen and to ensure that families felt supported through this entire process. We knew that each family would bring their own unique perspective of how their story had unfolded within our organization. As a team, it was important for us to hear their stories and to learn from their experiences. We also hoped that their perspectives could further define the strategy that would be developed for patients and families in the future.

We conducted two family focus groups, which were attended by 11 family members. All participants expressed their gratitude at being contacted and felt that this work was of the utmost importance. All said they would be open to being more involved at a future time. One family member shared, "The dying experience forged a lifelong connection for me with Sunnybrook and when I got the letter I thought, great, you didn't forget about us." This comment continues to resonate with the purpose of our work, constantly reminding us of the role we play in the stories of families, which do not end with the death of a loved one, but continue long after.

We learned from the family members that most had had positive experiences, but a few did not. They were impressed with the care they and their family members had received, were pleased by the respect for religious beliefs and lack of "agism," and spoke of the important role the palliative care team had made in their experiences. We learned that how we supported transitions in care was crucial, ensuring we maintained clear communication about what was happening, why it was happening, and helping them to know what to expect. Families remembered very clearly "bad communication" and could repeat phrases and words that they felt were not supportive or caring.

We also asked the family members to provide us with feedback on the identified domains of care to better understand if these were actually the areas of care that were most important for families. Additionally, they participated in a pilot of the new NRCC EOL Family Satisfaction tool. It was important for us to understand what it was like for families to complete the survey after losing a loved one. We wanted to know if they felt that the tool provided a vehicle to share their experience of care.

The family members did confirm that the domains identified in the literature were in fact the areas of care that were important to their experiences. After completing the new satisfaction tool, they also shared what it was like for them to do so, confirming that the questions in the survey would have provided them with the opportunity to give important feedback on the care they and their loved ones had received. Additionally, they spoke about how long after their loved ones had died when they thought it would have been best for them to receive the survey as grieving family members.

Participation in the focus groups with these families was a powerfully moving experience and we are so grateful to the families who returned to Sunnybrook, to open their hearts, so that we could learn. It also highlighted the imperative for us to find ways to stay connected with families for whom we have provided care. One family member shared that when she received the letter of invitation, she was so encouraged, as it told her that "they [Sunnybrook] had been remembered." Each family had a story to share. These stories were about people they loved, people who were and continue to be important to them. We had the privilege to hear about those individuals, their relationships, and their last moments of life. This is the heart of why "it matters."

FOUNDATION OF PERSON-CENTERED CARE

When we care for the dying, we are caring for the living. We are caring for those who lived lives long before we came to know them. It is our role to see them as "persons" first, to learn who they are and what is important to them. They are mothers, fathers, brothers, sisters, children, friends, and so much more. They have been connected to the world in ways far beyond our knowing. Recognizing the imperative of "knowing the person," the QDI is firmly built on the foundation of person-centered care. This philosophical approach ensures that care is respectful and responsive to individual preferences, needs, and values, and that these values guide clinical decision making. It means that we ask questions to learn what is most important and what matters to individuals, making intentional efforts to begin interactions from that perspective and to integrate those perspectives into all aspects of care through human connectedness.

When I think of why it matters, I think of my father, who passed away many years ago. I think of how important he was in my life and how he has shaped who I am today. I am grateful in ways that are difficult to describe with words, but experience through other ways. When my father died, we planted a black oak tree in his memory. The tree is minutes from my home, and on my morning jogs, I often run past his cemetery, and I think of him. I look at the sky and the clouds, and the geese by the cemetery pond, and I know he continues to be a part of me. It matters because as health care providers, we have the opportunity to enter into the lives of others, to see those individuals as people, to learn about who they are and the life they lived, because they will be remembered.

Knowing the person matters. Working as a nurse on a palliative care unit, it was very important to find ways to get to know the person. Patients and families were encouraged to bring in photos and personal items and to share stories that gave meaning and honor to their lives. Images of smiling faces, pets, gardens, and grandchildren stood guard, constantly reminding us of the person we were caring for. Favorite music and soft melodies danced in the air and down the hallways, often bringing back fond memories that were shared in quiet presence, during the middle of the night.

As health care providers, we have the special privilege to walk with others to the "edge of their life." I heard these words stated in a palliative care conference many years ago, and they continue to resonate within my being. I cannot remember who stated them, although I really wish I could, as they have significantly impacted my understanding of how important this work is. After a person's death, the family will leave the hospital and continue with their lives, and we continue on as health professionals to care for patients. We often do not know the experience of the family after the death of their loved one, how they will remember their experience at the hospital, and the role we played in their journey. I recently had the opportunity to meet a stranger, who shared her experience with me.

A CHANCE MEETING AT THE CEMETERY

It was Easter Sunday and I had gone to my father's cemetery to sit by his memory tree, planted in his honor, following his death. As I arrived, I noticed a woman sitting quietly in her car. As I walked to my father's black oak tree, I thought for a moment about how we were both there for our own reasons, with our own stories, on this Easter weekend. The branches of my father's tree were still barren from our long cold winter. The sun lay hidden behind a thin layer of clouds in the gray sky and seemed determined to demonstrate its brilliance on this day. The contrast of the glow from the hidden sun against the dark branches was beautiful to me and I moved backward taking a photo of the sky and the tree. It was at this moment that I met Melanie. I later learned, she had been visiting her mother's grave. As we stood in the cemetery sharing our stories, I learned that her mother had passed away almost a year ago following a stroke. She shared that she had made some very difficult decisions related to her mother's care. She had been told by a nurse that she was "courageous" for making these difficult decisions, but in reflection, was not certain what the nurse had meant by those words. Had her mother died as a result of these decisions? Would her mother have lived longer if she had made different decisions? Had she made the right decisions? I did share with Melanie that I was a nurse, and that I had worked in palliative care. We talked about the decisions that she had made. We did exchange numbers and later that evening I received at message from Melanie and she shared that her "spring of insight which lay dormant" since her mother's passing was reawakened.

After meeting Melanie, I had an ever-increasing awareness of how significant the moments are that we share with persons who are dying and their families. They are etched into the minds and hearts of those for whom we care. They will be remembered and it is imperative that we prepare ourselves as health care professionals to have these important discussions, because they matter.

EXPLORING OUR CONTEXT—FAMILY PERSPECTIVES

In a qualitative descriptive study that explored the experience of families who had lost loved ones through ovarian cancer, we learned about the importance of supporting families during this time (Das Gupta et al., 2008). Families shared their experiences describing how they felt, what helped them, and how they perceived caring.

▦ "We were extremely touched when, in the final hours, some of the health care team, you know, they'd come up after a 12-hour shift, and check on my mum, or give us a hug, which, having worked a lot of 12-hour shifts myself, I think it's really incredibly generous, because they didn't just run home, especially the night my mum was dying. I don't know how they knew—but they knew, and they'd come up, and they said good-bye to her, and gave us a hug. And I just thought that was really, really caring."

■ "You're filled with guilt no matter what you do. You know, you've done too much, you haven't done enough, did you do the right thing, did you say. . . you're always questioning yourself, And, although I felt positive about, you know, what I did for [loved one] and I know she appreciated it but you just always feel so stressed and so guilty."

■ "You almost start to feel, like for me anyways, this underlying anxiety. I'm usually, I'm a very together person, and sort of like this underlying— there was always like this underlying anxiety, I guess, is the best way to put it. There's nothing in between, like mum's having a good day, and you're like so happy, and then there's a bad thing, and then you're down. You just, you lose a sense of who you are, in that regard. . . but you just manage it. It was difficult, and it still is difficult."

Families discussed the importance of knowing what to expect and having information explained clearly and honestly. Some families described that it was often difficult to get information or answers from the health care team and that they had to work at it. They described this as a "tiring process," and that they sometimes "felt ignored." They shared that this came at a time, when they already felt "fatigued," "worn," and were living lives that had been turned "upside down."

■ "Like you know, you know we were getting ignored, you know. I would bug the nurses, 'how is mom today?' You know, they wouldn't come to us and tell us. Like if you want information you've got to ask, and ask, and ask."

■ "I came to my own conclusions. You know, nobody really explained it to us so I just thought it was, or you know, what was going to happen, like what happens to somebody in stage four, like what is failing, what is, what do they need, what to expect, what's coming next. I feel like we got none of that information at all."

And they talked about hope. . . .

■ "And you can't, you can't lose hope, there's always hope and try not to let people take it away. Although, you know, honestly, I would, I wouldn't say I was always like that every day for 3 years, but I was, I had to be on some level hopeful, or I'd probably would have just not been able to do all of the things that I was able to do. So I guess I still, I always found something to be happy about, or hopeful about."

Realizing that engaging in discussion with patients and families is so important to their experience, how prepared are staff to do this? In settings where EOL care is a primary focus of care, staff may feel more prepared to provide support. In clinical settings, where EOL care is not necessarily the primary focus, staff may be less comfortable and confident. These thoughts led us to explore the perspectives held by staff members about this topic.

EXPLORING OUR CONTEXT—STAFF PERSPECTIVES

In order to develop a full appreciation of our current context, we explored the experience of our interprofessional staff caring for persons who were dying using two methods. We conducted an organization-wide clinician survey and further engaged staff through focus groups.

The clinician survey served multiple purposes that included (1) raising organizational awareness as to importance of quality dying, (2) seeking staff perspectives related to competency and level of comfort with EOL care, (3) identifying local EOL initiatives and potential opportunities, (4) establishing baseline self-assessment of related skills, and (5) providing data to serve as a corporate indicator. Staff were invited to complete the survey through an organization-wide awareness-raising campaign called Let's Talk About It. Three hundred twenty-five staff members completed the survey with the greatest number of responses from nursing (60%). In the quantitative comments, 96% of staff agreed or strongly agreed that they viewed the quality of the dying experience to be just as important as the quality of any other care element provided in the hospital setting, 88% of staff stated that they were able to recognize when a patient was dying, and 76% of staff reported that they were comfortable both assessing the symptoms of a patient who is dying and discussing care elements unique to EOL care with dying patients. Staff members were passionate in their responses to the survey and illustrated their value of the topic through the many pages of written comments, where they provided descriptions of meaningful care, examples of challenges experienced when providing EOL care, and advocated for additional required resources to support that care. One respondent shared this:

> In North America dying is a taboo subject. Hospices barely exist in this culture, and yet they are by far the best way to die in Europe. Let's start by talking about what people want, how they want to die. Let's start by talking about the aggressive therapy we provide. Let's talk about resources and budgets. Let's talk about ethics. We need to begin the discussion first.

The clinician survey was followed by focus groups to explore the staff perspective in greater depth. Through a qualitative descriptive research study (Rivera & Das Gupta, 2013) three focus groups were held, each consisting of 5 to 10 interprofessional health care providers. Participants (*n* = 23) consisted of nurses, social workers, occupational therapists, physiotherapists, chaplains, and physicians from different medical/surgical wards. Approval from Sunnybrook's Research Ethics Board was achieved and these findings further informed the development of our strategy. The purpose of the focus groups was to explore and understand the experience of health care providers in giving EOL care, to identify system barriers and enablers, and to determine required staff support for the provision of the highest quality EOL care.

One important theme that emerged was "Transitioning Care." We heard from our teams of health care providers that there was an uncomfortable sense that care was "withdrawn" at the EOL. As care transitioned from active treatment to palliative care and comfort measures, core activities were reduced or stopped and roles of team members were changed or "discontinued." Nursing participants described a decreased frequency of assessment and monitoring, described as "taking off the monitors," "stopping vital signs," and "discontinuing labs." Patients were often moved to private rooms for privacy, curtains were drawn, and doors were closed. Staff felt that this left the perception for families that the care of their loved ones was less valuable.

One physiotherapist described that their professional role involves mobilizing patients. However, when a person's prognosis changes, their role also changes. Their involvement may be discontinued when rehabilitation is no longer the goal. They may continue to stay involved in the care through interventions such as chest physiotherapy or suctioning, when indicated. However, in most cases their services are discontinued. A second physiotherapist described the feeling of "taking a step back" or "backing off" from the care. They shared that this was often difficult for them, as they had developed important relationships with both the person and the family.

- "The thing is, it's supporting families and patients when they feel as though we've given up on them. From when they move from active treatment to palliative, they might feel that we are abandoning them."
- "Even things like monitoring, we stop taking vital signs, we stop monitoring, and the family, because they're used to seeing the monitors, used to seeing their loved one's heart rate, and then suddenly we're taking off those kind of monitors, it makes them wonder. We explain . . . I just say we are not monitoring those things anymore. I guess we have to find other ways to reassure them that the patients are comfortable."

Staff shared with us that they would like to feel better prepared to provide EOL care and did not feel that they had sufficient preparation through their education and training. They worried that they didn't have the "words" or "didn't know what to say," and in the absence of that, sometimes choose to not engage.

- "So, just off the top of my head I think, I began working in oncology about a year and a half ago. And I'd like to hear from other people as well, but um, there's no formal education, there's no formal training in how to do this . . . and I don't know what the expectation is that it's an innate skill or it isn't. I'm not sure but in my opinion, I think there's a big gap there. Um, so I think even maybe having that formal education and training and speaking to people who have the experience will be very very helpful."
- "And I don't even really know the basics. Some families ask, 'Oh, so what do I do now?' You know, about calling funeral homes. They don't even know where to start. So if we could give them a simple plan, 'Sorry, but this is what you need to do.' They have no idea. And you know, we need to give them something. Honestly, I have no idea either."
- "Um, I'm a nursing student right now. So I even noticed in going through the curriculum at school like they don't really touch on palliative care, death and dying and stuff like that. I feel like it's such an important thing and when we come in here, and then it's just, I don't know. It's such a new experience as for us as students. And you don't know how to deal with it. You don't know what to do for the patients either. You don't know how to react."
- "We should be having education more than once a year, because it happens every day because death happens every day. We can't be afraid of it."

These findings helped to clarify and define our first intervention, the Comfort Measures Strategy. It confirmed the need to approach EOL care from an interprofessional perspective, ensuring we clearly defined and articulated what care looked like and how it changed at the EOL. It also emphasized the need to include staff development, capacity building, and support. We recognized that we also needed to find a way to enhance our communication with families, and focus on how care *changes* at the EOL. It was at this point in time that we learned about the CARES tool. We felt that the tool provided the solution to ensure that there was an evidence-based approach to care that provided a framework and language for comfort assessment, education, communication, and overall care provided.

TAILORING KNOWLEDGE TO THE LOCAL CONTEXT—COMFORT MEASURES STRATEGY

The Comfort Measures Strategy is Sunnybrook's first intervention in the QDI, designed for broad implementation in our adult, acute care, inpatient setting. It can be defined as a multifaceted interprofessional strategy comprising a bundle of best practices aimed to improve the care of persons who are "imminently dying," defined as last days and hours.

The strategy specifically included the implementation of:

- Two evidence-based order sets
  - Comfort Measures Order Set incorporating the CARES model
  - No CPR Order Set

- Family resource materials
  - What to Expect in the Last Hours of Life
  - Coping With Death

- Capacity building for staff through coaching consultations provided by the PCCT

- Spiritual care consultation

- Eating for quality of life

- Integration into documentation and transfer of accountability

KNOWLEDGE TOOLS AND RESOURCES

The CARES tool has been integrated as a framework into clinical tools and processes including the Comfort Measures Order Set, Comfort Assessment, clinical documentation, and transfer of accountability (i.e., process for exchanging responsibility for a patient's care from one professional to another). The framework guides staff education and has additionally been used to restructure the clinician survey so that we can continue to evaluate comfort and confidence in providing EOL care. By embedding the framework into the supporting clinical tools and resources, we are guiding practice change by clarifying the desired behaviors, defining practice expectations, and making the information and knowledge available at the point of care.

The Comfort Measures Order Set is a core component of the Comfort Measures Strategy. It was developed to meet the specific care needs of persons who are "imminently dying," which means, within their last days and hours of life. The Comfort Measures Order Set is a structure that integrates evidence-based practices for (1) symptom management of most commonly experienced symptoms at the EOL, (2) comfort assessment, (3) patient/family education, and (4) interprofessional collaboration to support the holistic needs of patients and their families. The order set was developed by an interprofessional working group including stakeholders from the PCCT, nursing, pharmacy, spiritual care, and nutrition. The No CPR Order Set is embedded within the Comfort Measures Order Set, as is required in order to initiate "Comfort Measures."

The greatest challenge is to *not* view the order set as a checklist, or a one-dimensional list of interventions to support quality dying. It must be viewed as a representation of an organization's commitment to integrate quality dying into all that we do. The order set and all that it stands for must "live" within the organization. The selections are care processes that define "what" care is provided, noting that there are important interprofessional relationships that define "how" the care unfolds collaboratively in the clinical setting.

One selection item on the order set is "comfort assessment every 2 hours and as needed." The Comfort Assessment is a new clinical practice, framed using the CARES tool. It changes assessment from that of the traditional system assessment to better reflect the care needs of a dying person. Assessment descriptions and suggested interventions are preprinted on the back of the order set, as a readily accessible reference to further support clinical decision making. Nurses have also been given lanyard cards with summary points from the CARES tool to support practice in the moment and documentation of care provided.

PATIENT AND FAMILY INFORMATION SHARING

Helping families know what to expect is an important role that is the responsibility of all interprofessional team members. Two key family resource materials were created to support the Comfort Measures Strategy. The first resource is called "What to Expect in the Last Hours of Life." This resource was created in an effort to answer questions commonly asked by families at the EOL, in a clear, simple, easy-to-understand, yet comforting format. The second resource is called "Coping With Death." It is most commonly provided by spiritual care chaplains after a death. This resource focuses on the emotional impact of losing someone close and provides practical information about topics such as financial arrangements and funeral planning. Direction to provide the family resources is included in the order set. Orders are not required for this intervention. However, including this care element helps to promote consistency in practice, through a defined practice expectation.

The resources are well used by staff as tools to enter into conversations with families and to answer difficult questions. The desired goal is that health care providers will continue to develop enhanced expertise in effective communication and education skills. The resources have become the building block for health care professionals in opening the door to dialogue with patients and family members and to becoming increasingly comfortable discussing what to expect at the EOL.

IT TAKES A TEAM—INTERPROFESSIONAL CARE

The order set includes consultations to interprofessional team members. The Comfort Measures Strategy is based on the principles of interprofessional care. It recognizes the important contribution of different roles and interconnectedness of those individuals working collaboratively to enhance the patient and family experience. The care unfolds in the moment as each care provider engages with both their unique and shared role contributions. Important care processes, such as interprofessional care rounds and bullet rounds, help to ensure that the whole team is knowledgeable about the needs, wishes, and concerns of the individual and that the plan of care is based on the individual's priorities about what is most important to him or her as a person. Consultation to both the spiritual care and the PCCTs is automatic. The roles of each team are described in detail below.

SPIRITUAL CARE—GRACEFUL PASSAGES AND DIGNITY WHEN IT MATTERS MOST

The role of spiritual care is described first. Thank you to Anke Flohr, who is the professional leader for spiritual care, and Bill Ford, who is a chaplain, at Sunnybrook for their leadership in developing these practices and for eloquently sharing how it is lived in clinical care.

Whoever you are, wherever you are from, whatever tradition guides your way, there comes a time when we all need to be touched through the heart (Stillwater & Malkin, 2002).

The spiritual care phone rings: "This is Lenora, nurse on oncology. We need a chaplain. We have an automatic referral for the Comfort Measures Order Set for Mrs. Hudson in room 10, bed 2." The chaplain on-call, Carlos, assures Lenora that he will be coming ASAP. He asks a few screening questions over the phone and finds out that Mrs. Hudson seems confused and unresponsive at times. Her daughter, Dorothy, is at her side. Chaplain Carlos is on his way.

The Comfort Measures Order Set includes an automatic referral to spiritual care grounded in a model of care that is person/family centered and holistic in nature, addressing all needs and concerns relevant to care, including spiritual and religious ones. Person-centered spiritual care allows the beliefs, values, affiliations, and practices of the patient/family to be the basis upon which care is provided. The spiritual care providers (chaplains) respond promptly and in person. They explain the role of spiritual care on the interprofessional team to the patient and/or family, offer spiritual care (by consent), and address the spiritual needs of the dying patient and his or her family. Their approach is spiritually inclusive and respectful of each person's faith, traditions, or nontraditional beliefs—honoring the whole person by recognizing the relationship between mind, body, and spirit. Spirituality is an idiosyncratic and culturally diverse concept:

> Spirituality is the dynamic dimension of human life that relates to the way persons (individual and community) experience,

> express and/or seek meaning, purpose and transcendence, and the
> way they connect to the moment, to self, to others, to nature, to the
> significant and/or the sacred. (Nolan, Saltmarsh, & Leget, 2011)

Spiritual care is a core element of palliative care as defined by the World Health Organization (WHO, 2007). Spiritual issues become paramount at the EOL. The goal is to provide a compassionate presence, offer emotional support in the grieving process, and help the patient and/or family to explore their own spiritual concerns, issues, beliefs, values, and spiritual resources to assist in life's closure. Spiritual care providers assess the patient's spiritual history, practices and rituals, signs and symptoms of spiritual distress, and psychosocial–spiritual needs.

The importance of both religion and spirituality is that they provide a context in which people can address ultimate questions about the meaning of life, illness, and death; cope with their experiences; and find a sense of hope, inner harmony, and peacefulness in the midst of the existential challenges of life. If requested, the spiritual care team will facilitate rituals and religious services or involve clergy from the patient's religious community. In addition, chaplains provide information about next steps, including funeral planning and resources for bereavement support (booklet available "Coping with the Death of a Loved One—A Practical Guide for Family Members and Caregivers"). The chaplains document the meeting with the patient in the patient's chart, summarize the spiritual assessment, and outline the care and follow-up plan.

Chaplains are companions for the living and dying . . . touching hearts: Shortly after Chaplain Carlos had received the page from Nurse Lenora he arrived on the oncology unit. Lenora updated Carlos on Mrs. Hudson. Mrs. Hudson was 85 years old suffering from metastatic breast cancer. She had been admitted to the medical/radiation oncology unit for 2 weeks. Mrs. Hudson had a 2-year history of breast cancer and had been doing well prior to this admission. She lived in her own home and enjoyed a "reasonably good quality of life." Mrs. Hudson's condition had deteriorated significantly since she arrived on the unit and the interprofessional team had concerns that Mrs. Hudson may not be able to return to her home. Several members of the team had met with Mrs. Hudson's daughter, Dorothy, to address goals of care and it was decided that Mrs. Hudson would be transferred to the palliative care unit once a bed became available. As Mrs. Hudson waited for a bed in the palliative care unit, her condition continued to worsen and it became apparent that her death was approaching faster than anticipated.

The comfort measures order was initiated and that was when Chaplain Carlos was informed. When entering the room Carlos found Mrs. Hudson unresponsive with her daughter keeping vigil at the bedside. After obtaining consent for the visit, Chaplain Carlos was welcomed by Mrs. Hudson's daughter who was eager to speak at length about her mother.

Chaplain Carlos listened deeply as Dorothy spoke openly of how her father died when she was a young girl and how her mother, as a single parent, had lovingly raised her. She spoke of the challenges the death of her father had presented and how her mother was able to rise above the challenges and provide a "decent" life for them. She described how her mother had made sacrifices to ensure she was cared for and the many lessons her mother had taught her about living well. The chaplain engaged Dorothy to share the parts of her mother's life that she remembered most, especially those times when she sensed her mother was most alive. As if viewing a family photo album, Dorothy recalled stories that reflected her mother's work ethic, her unconditional love and family values, her sense of humor and her athletic ability—especially her love of curling and how she had curled even in her older years. Dorothy spoke of all that had given her mother meaning and purpose in life.

Chaplain Carlos inquired about roles that Mrs. Hudson had played in her life. Dorothy, without hesitation, spoke of the many roles her mother had played but none more important than how her mother had been both a mother and a father for her; naming her mother as her "rock." The chaplain provided a safe space for Dorothy to speak of her mother's many accomplishments and all that made her proud. In the midst of the interaction with the chaplain, hoping her mother could still hear, Dorothy held her mother in her arms and gave voice to all she wanted to say to her mother.

Chaplain Carlos explored Dorothy's own anticipated grief—and with that came the knowledge that Dorothy was the primary caregiver for her husband who was living with dementia; she was attempting to cope with her husband's failing health. She spoke of her unresolved grief of not being able to have children of her own; and the immense responsibility she felt of being an only child. Dorothy also realized that she was becoming an "adult orphan" and the grief and fear that she had bottled up inside her rose to the surface.

Chaplain Carlos also explored the role of faith and spirituality in her mother's life. Dorothy admitted that while faith was important to her mother, it was less so for her. Dorothy indicated her mother was a devout Roman Catholic who found comfort and strength from her faith and the rituals of her church. Dorothy also indicated that her mother had found a sense of community and belonging in her faith community. Exploring what her mother might want at this time, Carlos was able to facilitate a visit from the Roman Catholic priest for sacramental ministry, particularly sacrament of the sick. Chaplain Carlos also provided a booklet "Coping With the Death of a Loved One" to help prepare Dorothy for funeral planning and to further help as a guide for many of the practical details that would follow the death of a loved one.

The chaplain's role in this encounter was to provide emotional and spiritual support for Dorothy, to provide an opportunity for her to see the value in her mother's life, to review all that had given her mother purpose and meaning, and to provide a sense of dignity to this stage in the life journey. The chaplain allowed Dorothy to see that while her mother was actively dying, she was still alive and would continue to be so in her own life and memories. The chaplain provided grief support as Dorothy struggled with various losses and regrets in her life. The chaplain took the time to be present to Dorothy and to highlight how her mother had lived well and to further explore what would be required to allow her mother to die well.

When Mrs. Hudson died the next evening Chaplain Carlos was there with Dorothy saying the final good-bye.

> The depth of my grief is a constant with the breadth of my love.
> I would never sacrifice one to avoid the other. (Fumia, 2003)

EATING FOR QUALITY OF LIFE

Eating for quality of life is an aspect of comfort care we are continuing to develop. As we know, individuals with end-stage diseases, such as severe dementia and cancer, eat less as part of the natural progression of their disease. However, as we focus on quality dying, we are seeking to change the frame of mind around nutrition at the EOL. The goal is to promote quality of life, with the priority becoming comfort and meal enjoyment as opposed to maximizing and optimizing nutritional status. Dietitians and speech language pathologists play an important role in working with patients and families to achieve this goal. Katelynn, a dietitian, shares a personal reflection on her role and insights related to this important topic.

Mia

In the natural order of things, these would be exciting times for Mia. She would be graduating from university, enjoying the summer sun, and wondering what the world holds next for her. Instead, I remember her fondly and have faith that she is in a better place.

Mia was 21 years old when we first met. I was just a year older, freshly starting my career, and I felt connected to her vibrant spirit. Every time I would stop by to check in on her, she would tell me not to worry, that she was eating and drinking well, and that others needed me more. But as her chemotherapy became more aggressive, so did the side effects; the nausea and vomiting was unforgiving and intractable. IV nutrition followed, and during a daily review of her chart, four words stunned me: Failed third line chemo. This shining star (just a year younger than me!) had a prognosis of less than three months. My tears spotted the pages and it took all my strength to maintain composure during discussions about her care. Comfort care, including the withdrawal of IV nutrition, was decided. Mia wasn't hungry or thirsty, and the idea of drinking a supplement or forcing down a tray of food did not align with her definition of comfort. I was at a loss, how could I possibly ensure she was adequately nourished? When I turned to Mia, her answer was simple. "Just keep coming to visit me every day" she replied, "Maybe one day we can have a Big Mac together." And that's when I realized that it wasn't all about clinical skills, equations, and optimizing or maximizing nutritional intake, but quality of life at EOL. My perspective shifted to focus on Mia eating solely for the purpose of comfort and enjoyment. On one of our last days together, she had a few bites of a burger and a couple of fries, and I couldn't have been happier.

Katelynn Maniatis

PALLIATIVE CARE COACHING CONSULTATION

The PCCT is an interprofessional team including medicine, advanced practice nursing, and social work. The primary role of the team, in regard to the Comfort Measures Strategy, is to support professional development, capacity building, and skilled dialogue, in the moment, with health care providers. Their role is to help staff find ways to become as comfortable as possible with "being present" with families, when presence offers more value than words. Concerns expressed by families such as "he seems to be suffering," "her breathing looks difficult; she is gasping for air," "can't you give him more for pain?" "why is this taking so long; can you tell me when he will die?" often challenge staff. How does one respond to these comments or questions in a way that conveys compassion and caring? While there may be no right answers, we do need to become comfortable with these moments.

The PCCT works very closely with staff to build knowledge, skills, competence, comfort, and expertise in providing EOL care and having compassionate discussions with families at the EOL. Using guiding questions, and reflective practice, the team encourages staff to assess their own knowledge of the Comfort Measures Order Set and care interventions as they relate to the dying person's goals, priorities, and patient and family preferences. The coaching consultation builds on the existing strong relationship between palliative care and oncology. In addition to one-on-one dialogue regarding the care plan with staff caring for dying patients, a side-by-side patient comfort assessment and discussion with family is encouraged. These collaborative "in the moment" meetings of palliative care consultant, staff member, the patient, and family together focus on active listening and being therapeutically present, based on what is most important to the person and family. Sharing observations of the patient's comfort and how signs of discomfort are managed at the bedside in the presence of family communicates caring, builds staff confidence, and encourages family to participate. Staff use the newly developed family resource materials to guide the conversation and to additionally share changes the family may see as death approaches. They answer questions and sometimes remain present together in meaningful silence. All interactions are followed by an opportunity to reflect on the dialogue and learn from the experience. The goal is to become more aware of one's thinking and reasoning, including how they were feeling and gained insights. Staff at our organization have found these learning opportunities to be extremely important and helpful in developing not only greater comfort, but also a deeper self-awareness.

A specific example of how a side-by-side collaborative patient assessment builds confidence and competence in staff is as follows: A young woman with cancer was close to death. A large group of immediate and extended family was keeping a vigil at her bedside. Entering a patient's room under these circumstances can be anxiety provoking for inexperienced staff, who may be hesitant to engage in dialogue with the patient's family. The palliative care consultant and nurse entered the patient's room together and introduced themselves. The consultant stated their intention to assess the patient's comfort. "Would you like us all to leave?" asked the patient's husband. The family was invited to stay; this provided an opportunity for the consultant to explain what a comfort assessment involved and for the nurse to witness caring and compassionate communication with the family. The consultant and nurse observed the patient silently for a brief time. They spoke quietly with each other first, and then to the family about their findings. As they left the room, the patient's sister followed them into the hallway asking, "How much longer do you think it will be before she dies?" This question is often asked of the palliative care team; in this case the consultant turned to the nurse, encouraging her to respond. The nurse's willingness to respond to the question conveyed a desire to provide support and comfort and to continue engaging in dialogue with the family.

Pat Daines is an advanced practice nurse on the PCCT. She is also the professional development lead for the QDI and has provided the leadership for the Comfort Measures Strategy with a focus on staff development and reflective practice. We all have lessons to learn from our interactions with patients and families, and using reflective practice enables us to learn from our experiences and change our behavior for future interactions. Pat shares a personal insight in the following, followed by a team story. This is one of many examples of changes that have occurred through coaching consultation and building a culture that values "quality dying."

WHY AM I HERE?

I knew very little about T. She was 72 years old and was recently diagnosed with head and neck cancer. She was currently undergoing radiation therapy and was having increasing pain with this. My mission was to learn more about her pain and to offer some strategies to better manage it.

I felt quite confident that I could help her as I entered her room; how did things go so wrong? After introducing myself, I asked her about her pain. "Pain is pain" was all she said. Confused, but undaunted I continued to try to get her to tell me what I needed to know. "Why am I here?," was all she said. "I should be in Florida." It was ironic that she should say this as I was experiencing the same sentiment; "Why am I here?"

I did, however, follow her cue and asked about her reference to Florida. That was the beginning of our therapeutic, human connection. She shared stories with me of her active life, her passion for golf, and spending much of her winter in Florida with friends. She was struggling to come to terms with her cancer and how her life was changing. Being here in the hospital, in pain, was a constant reminder of what she was losing, and what might forever be lost.

I learned so much from caring for T. She has helped me to better understand the complexities of pain, and the concept of total pain. I often carry her with me in my thoughts as I enter a patient's room to help guide me to be present in the way I am most needed.

TAKING TIME TO KNOW WHAT IS MOST IMPORTANT

Getting to know the person we are caring for is important. Sometimes we learn about last wishes. Although the last wish of a dying person is not always possible, when it is, it is rewarding for everyone. I was caring for an elderly Muslim person who was dying. In the week that he was admitted to the hospital a very popular spiritual leader of his faith was coming to the Air Canada Centre, a large convention center in Toronto, Canada. Thousands of faithful followers were to come together to hear inspirational words of wisdom and faith. He had planned to be among the followers sharing and taking in the delightful messages. Unfortunately, he lay in a hospital bed waiting for his friends or family to visit so they could share what had been said; what they learned and heard. His wish that day was to have his bed turned to face Mecca, so that when his leader was giving his message, he could pray amid the believers. And knowing this wish, the nurses did their best to position his bed in the direction of Mecca. He prayed and was at peace that his prayer would be heard among the thousand others that day.

Kalli Stilos is also one of the advanced practice nurses on the PCCT. Here, she shares her experience about how the CARES model has supported her own clinical practice. This story describes important elements of the "Coaching Consultation" that are being shared and embedded into the clinical practice of all nurses.

WHAT DO YOU SEE?

As a palliative care advanced practice nurse, the CARES tool has been imprinted in my head and so when I'm asked to see someone in consult for EOL care, I use that simple framework to help guide my discussion with the family about what to expect as their loved one gets closer to death. Helping them understand the signs and symptoms is part of easing their anxiety during this time. I recently met a daughter who was very worried and unsettled watching the dying process of her elderly mother. Her mother was being cared for on a general internal medicine ward and that seemed to be adding to her distress. She had hoped that her mother would be cared for on a palliative care unit and was concerned that the nurses on this unit would not have the same skills. During my visit, I sat with her and walked her through my assessment using the CARES model. Each time I went through one of the components I asked her, "What do you see? Do you feel the same?" Caring side by side with family members, sharing what we are seeing and noticing, and enabling their perspective to lead the care is so important. This also helps me to discuss the various medications the nurses are administering for each of the symptoms that may be exhibited. I did this on a daily basis until her mother was transferred to the palliative care unit. It was such a relief for the daughter having more knowledge about the dying process. She knew what she should be watching for and, if she saw those symptoms, she could call the nurse and an intervention would be available.

Reflective practice provides the space to stop and think. Sooner or later we learn that life is like one ongoing conversation, revealed if we stop to listen. Antonio Machado has written that "The deepest words of the wise. . . . teach us the same as the whistle of the wind when it blows" (Machado & Bly, 1983).

Personally reflecting on "quiet presence," I know the moment I learned its impact, what it felt like, and how powerful it could be. I would like to share this story as one example of the ongoing conversation that lives within all of us.

My Uncle Lyall was a man who lived his life out loud. He didn't have children of his own and perhaps that was the reason he played such a large role in my life. He called me "Peanut." I remember the summer he told me that he had been diagnosed with lung cancer. We were at the cottage on vacation and I was 11 years old at the time. He told me he was having treatment for his cancer and he showed me the dots on his chest for his radiation therapy. At the time, I really didn't know what it all meant.

At Christmas time, when Uncle Lyall came to visit, I remember feeling stunned. He looked so different. He was so thin and his skin looked gray, hanging in deep wrinkles around his face. That evening there was much whispering and the tone was serious. After dinner, he took a short rest and I was asked to go wake him. As I stood at his side, I remember watching him sleep. I wondered if this is what people looked like when they had died. I didn't want him to die. He must have sensed me there and woke up, reaching for my hand. "Hey, Peanut" was all he said. He squeezed my hand for a very long time. Although he did not say one word, I felt like he said so much. He held me with his eyes, his heart, and his soul. And in this brief moment, when facing my greatest fear, I felt my heart smile.

CARING IS EVERYONE'S ROLE

A colleague of mine recently shared a story that she had been given by a wise elder when she lived in the South Pacific, and was very close with indigenous teachers. She shared that they taught her about a very special tapestry, an invisible shawl woven with compassion and love by the ancestors. This invisible shawl gently covers those in pain and grief to support them when they are hurting. She then shared her vision: "Imagine that a compassionate hospital is like that. It provides an invisible shawl of comfort and love for patients and families. People feel it and trust they are in good hands the moment they enter the hospital. This is a wonderful vision."

Creating a caring, compassionate culture is everyone's responsibility. Regardless of role, it is acknowledged that all team members contribute to the experience of "caring," which seeks to bring to life the metaphor of the invisible shawl. Interprofessional health care providers at Sunnybrook have described the significance of "caring" within their roles through a qualitative descriptive study that explored the meaning of caring within and among health care professionals providing cancer care (Das Gupta, Osmar, & Daley, 2009). This study included two phases. In phase one, six uniprofessional focus groups were held each with nurses, social workers, dietitians, pharmacists, physicians, and radiation therapists. In phase two, the findings were reviewed within two interprofessional focus groups, to discuss and explore related practice implications. From this study we learned that all health care professionals did view caring as integral to their roles, and a universal experience. They described the importance of emotional caring within their clinical practices as a means of attending to the moment and stillness, and how they used "self" and "presence" in caring interactions.

- "I think caring is a **universal experience** . . . at the end of the day, we are human beings here interacting with other human beings." (Physician)
- "**I don't think we experience it any different than in another profession**— the nurse, the physician. I think we come to the patient from a different vantage point because of our knowledge base and what we are taught in terms of medications but ultimately, it is about caring for the patient and their experience." (Pharmacist)
- "The **true presence** of being with people." (Nurse)
- "There are times when people need us in a very non specific way, in a way that they can't articulate. They may not have a particular concrete need . . . but what they need is that caring, sort of hand holding . . . just **literally being there** to accompany them through." (Social worker)

We are seeing and hearing examples of how caring is lived within our organization every day, and these stories are increasingly being shared. This is one example. At the Professional Council for Social Workers, the Comfort Measures Strategy was being highlighted, with an overview of the available tools and resources to support practice. The social worker who was active in the pilot implementation brought meaning to the strategy, tools, and resources by sharing a story from her practice. She described how she had cared for man who was living with intolerable pain who wanted to die. He was continuously calling out loudly, and the team was unsure about how to best meet his needs. She shared that when she first introduced herself, the man was not interested in interaction. She remained in quiet presence with him and slowly began to ask him simple questions about his interests and who he was as a person. She learned that he was retired and since his retirement he had enjoyed golfing.

Unfortunately, he was no longer able to do this. He went on to talk about his favorite golfing moments and soon came to the realization that these moments were lived when he golfed with his daughter. He shared that golfing had given them a common interest they could enjoy together as father and daughter, even if few words were shared. Through the dialogue he found comfort in the easy conversation, gained new insight, and felt his pain ease.

CARES—"S" STANDS FOR SELF-CARE

In this same study, staff also discussed the experience of caring as having unintended consequences, which were often described as the burden of caring, impacting them both emotionally and professionally.

- "You go home not so much physically exhausted . . . but emotionally. You find yourself mentally exhausted because you give so much all the time. And it impacts your personal life." (Nurse)
- "Whatever their needs are you are constantly taking care of them and they are like draining your resource both mentally as well as physically. You try to juggle the workplace as well as what is going on in your family, so that in the end of it, sometimes a simple thing like in my household every time when there are peaches or apples I am the one who is eating the bruised or rotten one . . . so you are kind of suffering wondering, when I am going to get the fruit that is perfect?" (Pharmacist)

I know these pressures very well and have experienced them personally. I know what it feels like to care for individuals and to feel the weight of that caring. I can remember so very clearly working on a medical radiation oncology patient care unit, where we had experienced a number of deaths in a very short period of time. I remember one night when I was caring for a young man. His wife was drained, but wanted to stay the night. She knew her husband was dying and could not bring herself to sleep in his room. She slept on a cot in the sunroom and asked that I wake her when "it was time." As her husband's death drew near, I woke her. She knew what "waking" meant. She wrapped her arms around me and cried quietly, asking over and over again, "What will I do with his clothes?" I had no words. I only held her. I continued to think of her and her husband long after my shift. I thought of the other patients and families I had cared for and had gotten to know. I felt the burden of caring. I have seen that repeated losses can have an impact, and that caring for one's "self" and "each other" is a priority. Through ongoing discussions with staff, we know that these are concerns about the burdens or stresses of caring that must be heard and recognized. The following concerns were identified when exploring the experience of interprofessional staff providing EOL care.

- If we want to find ways to better support patients and families . . . we also need to find ways to support staff who provide this care.
- "I think in terms of what we do well is indeed caring for patients and their families. What I would say that we don't do so well is caring for the staff afterwards . . . I don't know if we actually acknowledge the effect death has on people working in health care."

Although caring can provide great personal and professional satisfaction, when the unintended consequences are not addressed, and are additionally complicated by further organizational pressures, both quality care and quality work life for staff can become compromised. This is an area that we are continuing to explore and develop after exploring the "experience of health care providers," we have now embarked on a second study, to better understand what "specific self-care support" measures would be of greatest assistance to staff. These results have not yet been analyzed, but will inform a specific strategy for staff support.

We realize that for staff to provide care for patients and families, it is our organizational responsibility to provide access to formal and informal support. We consistently share the message that the "S" in the CARES model stands for self-care, and is an essential element of all patient care. We highlight currently available supports: unit-based debrief sessions; formal support from spiritual care, social work, and the palliative care consultation team; informal support from colleagues and team members; our corporate memorial service; and Sunnybrook staff wellness programs (e.g., fitness gym, exercise classes, yoga, pilates, Zumba, reflexology, massage therapy, Nordic pole walking) and our employee assistance program. We encourage staff to pay attention to how they are feeling, and to talk about how they are doing and what they need to help them continue caring. We begin sharing this message in orientation, as staff enter our organization, and hope that this message creates a safe space for staff to openly talk about self-care.

REAL PRESSURES . . . WHERE DO WE GO FROM HERE?

As an organization, we have found ourselves co-creating the story of quality dying. We listened to the voices of the persons we were caring for to learn what is most important to them, we designed a multifaceted strategy that not only embeds evidence into our daily clinical processes, but also supports staff to build competency for skilled dialogue and communication. But as we listened to the voices of our staff, we heard the real challenges and struggles that exist for them when caring for individuals who are dying, most notably, in the acute care setting. Our study revealed that there are multiple competing time pressures, space pressures, and a perceived lack of appreciation for the equal value of meaningful dialogue and technical care. Staff find themselves forced to balance the needs and expectations of the acute care setting, often presenting barriers for meeting the needs of dying patients and families, including even what might appear to be basic needs such as providing a "comfortable space for dying" that is "peaceful" and "quiet" or even finding a space to engage in an important conversation.

SPACE

- "You know, we're not a palliative care unit but we're almost anyways an extension of the palliative care unit. And so, we're providing the space that's comfortable for patients to die peacefully. And even in every single room, there's a PA system. A dying patient is subjected to a voice every two seconds. For someone to answer the phone or for someone to go to the certain room."
- "We don't have a quiet space. Especially in the day, you can't find a chair, never mind a room. Umm, right? I mean it's really a standing-room-only in the hallway to discuss everything, thank you very much. It isn't really very difficult, with the physical space."

TIME

Staff described that the atmosphere of the units was often not conducive to a peaceful death, as they were busy and noisy. The surgical floors were fast paced with high patient turnover. Staff reported that they felt pressured to have sufficient time to provide comfort and care to both patients and families.

- "But at the same time, we know the confines of what we have to work within and so it's tough as a professional, but as a human being, to try to be able to support and hear what the families are saying, and you completely agree with what they are saying, but it feels like there's nothing you can do about it. So how do you deal with that? So you kind of come across as being, um um, almost, I don't want to say not caring, but sometimes I think that the families feel that we're not very helpful because we can't make those changes; that we can't solve every problem."
- "In that it's so busy, it's noisy, and also so many things are going on. So I find sometimes, we may try to do our best, but it's not. [Because] of the atmosphere. And there may be three patients in a room. One's dying and

the other two are feeling sad also. They don't know this other one person. But I find that it's really not conducive to a peaceful death and dying."

Nurses in particular reported feeling rushed with multiple responsibilities. They stated that they wanted to spend the time with patients and their families but found themselves unable to do so.

- "Often I feel that we are so rushed, just, you know, dealing—especially if we're going to give chemotherapy or something like that. Your focus is on that and it's hard to find the time to spend with the family that you want to see. You want to spend enough time, but you can't."

Staff also reported that the rapid patient turnover and flow of patients within the system were experienced as the need to move patients "in and out." It prevented them from providing support even after a patient dies.

- "Providing the emotional support to dying patients and their families doesn't seem to be viewed as important, say, as to giving chemo or doing something else, right? And I think, there's pressure, like I think someone else was saying. As soon as one patient dies, then you're on, you have to be on to the next. And I think it's a real reality. It's a real pressure. But maybe even changing the culture, in such a way that says, this is my designated time to do this. But there is so much pressure in getting patients moving in and out, in and out, in and out, in and out, from like higher levels that, um, that time doesn't exist always. Because you have to be moving on to other things that have to be done as opposed to things that are nice to be able to do."

EVALUATING THE CHANGE

We have developed an evaluation strategy to assist in measuring the impact of change related to the Comfort Measures Strategy. As shared earlier, we have created and implemented a Family Experience End-of-Life Survey, administered through NRCC. We receive quarterly results and our Quality Dying Steering Committee is accountable to provide oversight for reviewing our performance data. Based on the implementation strategy, we have identified key metrics, including process and outcome measures, which we are continuing to observe for trends of improvement. These have been provided for your interest. Additionally, the survey includes verbatim comments that are very important for our team to review as they include the voice of the patient and family and reflect the quality of the experience. We are very pleased to see early trends in improvement. We will continue to track these indicators very closely as they relate to the

Comfort Measures Strategy through the implementation of further strategies that target different components along the quality dying continuum of care (see Table 23.1).

TABLE 23.1
End-of-Life Care Satisfaction Survey

Overall satisfaction	Percentage positive score: "Overall satisfaction with end-of-life care."
Pain and symptom management	Percentage positive score: Did your family member receive too much or too little or just the right amount of medication for his or her pain?
	Percentage positive score: Did the staff who cared for him or her tell you about how his or her pain would be treated in a way you could understand?
	Percentage positive score: Did your family member have trouble breathing?
	Percentage positive score: How much help in dealing with his or her breathing did your family member receive?
Information to prepare family for approaching death	Percentage positive score: At any point during the admission, were you and/or your family member told that the outcome of this hospital stay was likely to be death?
	Percentage positive score: Did you or your family member receive any information about the medicines that would be used to manage his or her pain, shortness of breath, or other symptoms?
	Percentage positive score: Did you or your family member receive any information about what to expect while he or she was dying?
	Percentage positive score: Would you have wanted more information about what to expect while your family member was dying?
Standard order compliance	Percentage of eligible patients with completed NO CPR. Percentage of eligible patients with Comfort Measures Order Set.
	Mean number of hours prior to death where orders were completed.
Comfort measures assessments	Percentage of dying patients who receive the Comfort Measures Assessments (using the CARES model) every 2 hours and as needed—per the standard orders.

(continued)

TABLE 23.1
End-of-Life Care Satisfaction Survey *(continued)*

Palliative care consult team (PCCT) engagement	Percentage of dying patients who received a PCCT consultation.
	Percentage of dying patients who received a spiritual care consultation.
Staff education	Number of staff who completed the professional development learning module.

ORGANIZATIONAL CAPACITY AND INFRASTRUCTURE—BEST PRACTICE MATTERS

It is hard to imagine what can be accomplished when a group of passionate individuals put their minds and hearts together. Synergies are often created and new opportunities present themselves. This has occurred with our QDI. Sunnybrook has been recognized as a Best Practice Spotlight Organization (BPSO) candidate through the Registered Nurses Association of Ontario (RNAO). This means that we have entered into a 3-year partnership with RNAO to implement best practice guidelines (BPGs). During this formal partnership, our organization is required to select, implement, and evaluate BPGs that will have the greatest impact on patient care and outcomes. Following successful completion of the partnership, our organization will transition from candidacy to BPSO designation. This designation is similar to the Magnet Hospital Designation awarded in the United States. As part of our candidacy, we decided to implement the BPG "End-of-Life Care During the Last Days and Hours" (RNAO, 2011). The recommendations associated with the guidelines were inherent components of our Comfort Measures Strategy and included understanding common signs and symptoms present during the last days and hours of life; being knowledgeable about pain and symptom management intervention to enable individualized care; and planning, educating, and sharing information with individuals and families regarding potential symptoms and physical signs of impending death.

We have created a best practice implementation infrastructure called Best Practice Matters. The infrastructure is composed of a large network of interprofessional champions, called iLead Champions. The champions are frontline leaders who are aligned to priority best practices, of which quality dying is one. A "puzzle piece" image identifies the core best practices and clearly illustrates that person-centered care is in the center as the foundation of all care (see Figure 23.1).

iLead Champions, with a defined role profile, are educated in quality improvement and change management, through a program called iLead

FIGURE 23.1 Patient-centered care logo.

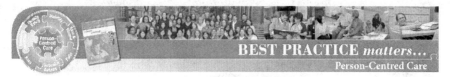

Foundations. This program was developed and is led by our quality and patient safety team. During each course, Champions are additionally prepared to provide local leadership for their specified best practice. iLead plays a key role in best practice implementation within their clinical setting by modeling excellence, influencing behavior change, identifying enablers and barriers, and leading discussion practice change through review of performance metrics. They continue to be developed and supported to fulfill these roles by middle leaders including patient care managers, advanced practice nurses, professional leaders, and clinical educators.

Champions are brought together monthly in "iLead Champions Connect" forums to discuss the practices they are implementing, to share the successes they are experiencing, and to brainstorm solutions to local challenges. The Champions have generated an energy and enthusiasm for change that cannot be described. As the practice implementation is rooted in quality improvement, the discussions have a strong data component. Performance data are shared with the staff and three key questions are explored:

1. What are the data telling us?
2. How are we moving toward the target?
3. What do we need to do to keep improving?

The Champions are the individuals who live the clinical experience and current context. They are the best ones to navigate the challenges and pressures; to find innovative, creative solutions; and to find ways to sustain those gains over time.

WHAT ARE WE SEEING, HEARING, AND NOTICING?

"Let's talk about it" is the phrase that we have chosen to highlight the QDI at Sunnybrook. We purposefully chose this phrase as it represents the social change that we would like to see and make happen related to death and dying. We would like to see everyone "talking about it." This means that in our general lexicon we develop a sense of comfort with speaking about death, that we recognize death is a natural life event, and that we consistently have important conversations with patients and families regarding their hopes, wishes, and preferences.

What happens when you start talking about death in your personal life? Conversations about death, dying, decisions, and memories become easier. In my own home, we have always tried to speak openly about these topics. We keep special people we have lost close to our hearts and we honor their lives with the stories we tell. When our family dog, Angel, passed away, my daughter Danae wrote a letter to her. Her letter tells me that despite her loss, she is comfortable.

> To Angel
>
> You were an amazing dog and I will always love you no matter what. Waking up every morning to the thought of you not being here is heart breaking, but I know you are now in a better place with Omi, Opa, Kazen, and everyone else. You will always be in our hearts no matter how close or far away you are. I will always remember our walks to the park, our trip to the cottage, and all of our other great memories together. I will now wake up every morning to the thought of you being very healthy and still the happiest dog. I love you Angel.
>
> Danae Das Gupta, 12 years old

What happens when you "talk about it" socially? It is very interesting to see what happens. I have found that surprisingly, people do not shy away from the topic. It is as though they feel relieved to be able to talk about the "elephant in the room," and they begin to share their stories. One winter evening, while out with a running group, the topic came up. I can't say I remember exactly how; likely related to a question about my job. But there we were, running and discussing the importance of quality dying. My running mate shared that she had recently become a hospice volunteer and described the value and meaning that it had added to her life. She later shared a story with me about a time she had accompanied a person she was caring for to the park. While they were there, enjoying the simplicity of the outdoor setting, a young child ran up to them, placing small yellow flowers on the arm of the person's wheelchair. It was a special moment, a moment about life and enjoying the beauty of the park together.

What happens when you "talk about it" in the workplace, in staff forums, and in hallway conversations? Wonderful things happen! Staff members pop by your office to share a story about themselves or a person for whom they have cared. They ask to meet with you to talk more about their experiences, what they are doing, how they are feeling about it, and their ideas for what else they could be doing. Staff members send e-mail messages, sharing words of hope and wisdom from both their personal and professional lives.

Some staff share their vulnerabilities about openly discussing how they don't feel prepared to care for those who are dying, because in their clinical areas, few people die. They tell you that when a patient dies, they feel distressed. They describe how they are not ready to be alone with a person after they have died and need to find another colleague to be present in the room with them as they prepare a body. They begin to brainstorm ideas about how they can become more comfortable and what their role might be in facilitating their team members to also discuss death and dying.

Staff begin to share resources with each other, including articles that are a "must read," videos that are a "must see," and websites that offer valuable resources. And they inspire me and everyone along the way. What are we seeing, hearing, and noticing? Change! Anecdotal, yes, you are correct. But in a complex adaptive system, these are patterns that are emerging, connecting, and generating continued energy and enthusiasm. We are still at the beginning of our story. We have carved off only a small piece of quality dying, being EOL care. But it is a start, a great start. Our staff are the magic and they are leading change. With the right tools and support, we look forward to the next chapter of our story.

REFERENCES

Bate, S. P. (2004). The role of stories and storytelling in organization change efforts. A field study of an emerging "community of practice" within the UK National Health Service. In B. Hurwitz, T. Greenlagh, & V. Sluktans (Eds.), *Narrative research in health and illness*. Oxford, UK: Blackwell.

Canadian Health Care Evaluation Project. (2010). Retrieved from http://www .virtualhospice.ca/en_US/Main+Site+Navigation/Home/For +Professionals/For+Professionals/Tools+for+Practice/Assessment+tools /CANHELP+(Canadian+Health+Care+Evaluation+Project)+Questionaire .aspx

Das Gupta, T., Moura, S., Fitch, M., Sapsford, M., Faltl, L., & Stilos, K. (2008). Qualitative exploration of families' experiences caring for loved ones with advanced ovarian cancer. Practice Based Research Grant, Sunnybrook Health Sciences Centre.

Das Gupta, T., Osmar, K., & Daley, A. (2009). Exploring the meanings of caring among health care professionals providing cancer care. Practice Based Research Grant, Sunnybrook Health Sciences Centre.

Estabrooks, C. A., Wallin, L., & Milner, M. (2003). Measuring knowledge utilization in health care. *International Journal of Policy Evaluation and Management, 1*, 3–36.

Fumia, M. (2003). *Safe passage—Words to help the grieving.* San Francisco, CA: Conari Press.

Machado, A., & Bly, R. (1983). *Times alone. Selected poems of Antonio Machado.* Middletown, CT: Wesleyan University Press.

Nolan, S., Saltmarsh, P., & Leget, C. (2011). Spiritual care in palliative care: Working towards an EAPC task force. *European Journal of Palliative Care, 18*(2), 86–89.

Pausch, R., & Zaslow, J. (2008). *The last lecture.* New York, NY: Hyperion Books.

Registered Nurses Association of Ontario. (2011, September). End-of-life care during the last days and hours. Best Practice Guideline. Ontario, Canada: Author.

Remen, R. N. (2006). *Kitchen table wisdom: Stories that heal.* New York, NY: Riverhead Books, the Penguin Group.

Rivera, R., & DasGupta, T. (2013). Exploring the experience of interprofessional health care providers. Canadian Hospice Palliative Care Conference, Ottawa, Canada.

Stillwater, M., & Malkin, G. (2002). Grace in practice: A clinical application guide for graceful passages, 20. Retrieved from http://www.leben-sterben.de/graceful_passages_en.PDF

World Health Organization (WHO). (2007). New guide on palliative care services for people living with advanced cancer. Retrieved from http://www.who.int/mediacentre/news/notes/2007/np31/en

Zimmerman, B., Lindberg, C., & Plsek, P. (1998). *Edgeware: Insights from complexity science for health care leaders.* Irving, TX: VHA Inc.

PART VII

Conclusions and Resources

CHAPTER 24

Summary of Steven's Peaceful Death

Care of the dying and their families requires a complex set of skills and understanding. Education, experience, and self-awareness are considered fundamental to providing quality evidence-based care. Other essential components identified by the literature review were incorporated into the CARES tool such as the need for communication, symptom management of pain, dyspnea, and terminal delirium, providing holistic supportive care that addresses the emotional, spiritual, and psychosocial needs of the dying patient and that promotes self-transcendence and the need for self-care.

The use of the CARES tool was discussed and demonstrated throughout this book through the exploration of Steven's active dying process. The theoretical foundation of the CARES tool, Self-Transcendence by Pamela Reed (2008), was adhered to as Steven's family was made to feel Steven's and their needs were being heard and acted on, that they were being viewed with respect, treated with dignity, and valued and cared for by the health care staff. These are the holistic tools necessary to help Steven's family transcend their emotional suffering and obtain closure. Their grief was supported and resources were provided that were patient specific, compassionate, and drawn from the very sense of humanity possessed by the health care provider.

The CARES tool helped guide the nursing staff's desire to provide quality end-of-life care for Steven and his family. They were assisted on how to address evidence-based common symptom management needs for Steven and provided suggestions to assist Steven's family both emotionally and spiritually. The nurses were also reminded to explore any personal bias that may impact their care. The CARES tool prompted the nurses to address the holistic needs of Steven and his family and identify supportive needs of the nurses.

The following is a summary of the care provided to Steven and his family based on the CARES tool.

1. Comfort: Steven's parents were encouraged to discard their isolation garb and hold their son. The order for protective isolation was cancelled as was the routine lab draws, the oxygen saturation and EKG monitor alarms, the hourly vital signs, and the standard hourly turning and repositioning. Steven's mother was encouraged to ask if she felt Steven needed to be turned or to request any other physical comfort measures.

2. Airway: Steven was actively dying and his respirations appeared agonal. The parents were informed his breathing at this point was involuntary and Steven was not suffering. The bi-pap was discussed as the increased pressure delivered to Steven's lungs was causing his upper body to make arch-like spasms with each forced breath. The need to reduce the pressure was discussed to minimize the chest wall spasm-like movements that could be uncomfortable for Steven. This was explored knowing the reduction in pressure delivery would reduce the amount of oxygen being delivered to Steven. A physical assessment of Steven noted bilateral fixed and dilated pupils, loss of gag and corneal reflexes, and no spontaneous movement to pain or to command. No adjustment in Steven's oxygen levels would prevent Steven from dying. The parents were helped to understand keeping the bi-pap at its current settings was only going to prolong Steven's dying process. The parents opted to reduce the bi-pap pressure and to increase the morphine continuous infusion to 2 mg an hour to ensure Steven was not suffering. The mother opted to use a tonsil suction and to frequently orally suction her son who was producing copious oral secretions. Steven developed a loud gurgling oropharyngeal rattle that was reduced with the administration of IV glycopyrrolate 0.4 mg every 15 minutes as needed. After three doses, the excess oral secretions were controlled. Steven's respirations were becoming less labored with increasing episodes of apnea. The parents were reminded that this was common in the dying process and the nurse caring for Steven remained in the room with Steven's parents.

3. Restlessness and delirium: Steven had progressed beyond the presence of delirium in his dying process. Hypoactive delirium could be present but given the absence of any reflexes and pupillary responses it would not be necessary to treat. No benefit would be derived from a trial of antipsychotics, and morphine was currently infusing for Steven's respiratory distress. No evidence of pain was present.

4. Emotional and spiritual support: The parents were asked if they needed anything. Coffee and water were brought to the room. A nurse sat in silence with the parents as each held their son's hand and took turns speaking softly to him. The father began to speak of his son. He shared that he wanted to become a nurse, of his love of the ocean, and back rubs. The mother began to cry softly when she shared her regrets at never again giving her son a back rub. It was

suggested she could give her son one now and the mother responded positively to the suggestion. Steven was positioned on his side as his mother lay next to him in his bed. His head was gently placed on the mother's shoulder as she draped her arm around his shoulders and began to massage Steven's neck and upper back. Steven's mother gently cried as she spoke to her son and continued to rub his back. The father placed his hand on his son's lower back and gently massaged the area. Their gentle crying continued and each was given tissues. The nurse asked if they were okay and if they would like some privacy. Both parents nodded yes and continued to hold their son close. A nurse checked on them frequently. Steven's respirations were almost nonexistent. Steven's mother began to sing softly to him and rock him as she must have done when he was a child. Steven stopped breathing and died in his mother's arms with his father at his side. The parents bravely told us that their son had died as a group of nurses remained outside Steven's room. Steven's death was confirmed by one of the nurses and the family requested some time alone with their son.

5. Self-care: The nurses outside Steven's room now numbered eight. All were teary eyed and two needed to leave the group and walk outside. Nicole, the social worker, remained from the start of Steven's final journey, and along with a spiritual care chaplain, sat with the nurses after they spent some time with the family. Nurses began to share their memories of Steven through their tears. Their professional grief was supported and they were reminded of the wonderful job they did in helping Steven and his family through this final journey. Steven had a loving and supported death surrounded by persons who loved and cared about him.

CONCLUSION

It is hoped that the CARES tool increases health care providers' awareness of the extensive and unique needs of the dying and the family. The skills required are not complex or high tech. They remain challenging because they require professionals to feel and be human, to be compassionate, empathize, and to be advocates.

There is an urgency to promote a change in health care in this country as the population continues to age. The curative focus of health care must be tempered with an acceptance of the need for compassionate, empathic, evidence-based end-of-life care. Comfort and quality of life must have a respected place in health care culture. Death should only be viewed as a failure by health care providers if the patient and family are allowed to suffer. The extensive knowledge available on care of the dying can prevent suffering during the dying process, but this knowledge has yet to be made a standard of care. The CARES tool is an attempt to bridge this gap.

The focus of the CARES tool is summarized best by two quotes that can be found printed on the border of the tool:

1. "There are worse things than having someone you love die. Most basic, there is having the person you love die badly, suffering as he or she dies. Worse still is realizing later on that much of his or her suffering was unnecessary" (Byock, 2012).

2. "It is the power of our own humanity that can make a difference in the lives of others. We must value this as highly as our own expertise" (Puchalski & Ferrell, 2010).

REFERENCES

Byock, I. (2012). *The best care possible: A physician's quest to transform care through end of life.* New York, NY: Avery.

Puchalski, C. M., & Ferrell, B. R. (2010). *Making health care whole: Integrating spirituality into patient care.* West Conshohocken, PA: Templeton Press.

Reed, P. G. (2008). Theory of self-transcendence. In M. J. Smith & P. R. Liehr (Eds.), *Middle range theory for nursing* (2nd ed., pp. 163–200). New York, NY: Springer Publishing.

CHAPTER 25

Recommended Learning Resources for Care of the Dying

END-OF-LIFE NURSING EDUCATION CONSORTIUM

Throughout this book the End-of-Life Nursing Education Consortium (ELNEC) program was frequently referenced. It is a national end-of-life educational program administered by the City of Hope (COH) and the American Association of Colleges of Nursing (AACN) and was developed to educate nurses on evidence-based hospice and palliative care. The ELNEC project was originally funded by a grant from the Robert Wood Johnson Foundation with additional support from the Aetna Foundation, Archstone Foundation, California HealthCare Foundation, Cambia Health Foundation, Milbank Foundation for Rehabilitation, National Cancer Institute, Oncology Nursing Foundation, Open Society Institute/Foundation, and the U.S. Department of Veterans Affairs. To learn more about the ELNEC project and their upcoming schedule of classes, go to www.aacn.nche.edu/ELNEC.

CITY OF HOPE PAIN & PALLIATIVE CARE RESOURCE CENTER

The City of Hope (COH) National Medical Center in Duarte, California, established an online resource for reference and education materials on palliative care in 1995 called the City of Hope Pain & Palliative Care Resource Center (COHPPRC). It acts like a clearinghouse to provide information and resources to improve pain management and palliative care. The COHPPRC supplies a variety of materials including pain assessment tools, patient education materials, quality assurance materials, research instruments, and other resources free of charge.

The available materials are organized into the following categories:

- Quality of life and cancer survivorship
- Spirituality
- Palliative care/end of life/bereavement
- Pain and symptom management approaches
- Special populations
- Education
- Quality improvement
- Ethical and legal issues
- Research instruments/resources
- Other resources: related organizations and websites

The COHPPRC can be accessed at http://prc.coh.org.

SUGGESTED READING FOR CULTURAL INFLUENCES ON END-OF-LIFE CARE

Ando, M., Morita, T., Ahn, S. H., Marquez-Wong, F., & Ide, S. (2009). International comparison study on the primary concerns of terminally ill cancer patients in short-term life review interviews among Japanese, Koreans, and Americans. *Palliative and Supportive Care, 7,* 349–355.

Doolen, J., & York, N. L. (2007). Cultural differences with end-of-life care in the critical care unit. *Demensions of Critical Care Nursing, 26*(5), 194–198.

Duke, G. (2013). Attitudes regarding life-sustaining measures in people born in Japan, China, and Vietnam and living in Texas. *International Journal of Palliative Nursing, 19*(2), 76–83.

Hosparus of Barren River, Central Kentucky, Lousiville, and Southern Indiana. (2009). *Cultural diversity in America: How different cultures approach end of life issues.* Louisville, KY: Hosparus.

Johnson, R., Newby, L. K., Granger, C. B., Cook, W. A., Peterson, E. D., Echols, M., Bride, W., & Granger, B. B. (2010). Differences in level of care at the end of life according to race. *American Journal of Critical Care, 19*(2), 335–343.

Koenig, B. A., & Gates-Williams, J. (1992). Understanding cultural difference in caring for dying patients. *Western Journal of Medicine, "Cross-cultural Medicine—A Decade Later," 157,* 247–374.

Robben, A. C. (Ed.). (2004). *Death, mourning and burial: A cross-cultural reader.* Malden, MA: Blackwell.

FURTHER READING

Gardiner, C., Gott, M., Ingleton, C., Hughes, P., Winslow, M., & Bennett, M. I. (2012). Attitudes of healthcare professionals to opioid prescribing in end-of-life care: A qualitative focus group study. *Journal of Pain and Symptom Management, 44,* 206–214.

Kerr, C. W., Donnelly, J. P., Wright, S. T., Luczkiewicz, D. L., McKenzie, K. J., Hang, P. C., & Kuszczak, S. M. (2013). Progression of delirium in advanced illness: A multivariate model of caregiver and clinician perspectives. *Journal of Palliative Medicine, 16,* 768–773.

Kirkpatrick, D. L., & Kirkpatrick, J. D. (2006). *Evaluating training programs: The four levels* (3rd ed.). San Francisco, CA: Berrett-Koehler.

Le, B. H. C., & Watt, J. N. (2010). Care of the dying in Australia's busiest hospital: Benefits of palliative care consultation and methods to enhance access. *Journal of Palliative Medicine, 13*(7), 855–860. doi: 10.1089/jpm.2009.0339

Long, J., & Perry, P. (2010). *Evidence of afterlife: The science of near death experiences.* [Kindle Fire version].

National Consensus Project (NCP). (2013). *Clinical practice guidelines for quality palliative care.* Pittsburgh, PA: National Consensus Project for Quality Palliative Care.

National Partnership for Action to End Health Disparities (NPA) (2011). National Stakeholder Strategy for Achieving Health Equity [Online Report]. Rockville, MD: U.S. Department of Health and Human Services, Office of Minority Health. Retrieved from http://www.minorityhealth.hhs.gov/npa/templates/content.aspx?lvl=1&lvlid=33&ID=286

Neuberger, J. (2013). *Independent review of the Liverpool Care Pathway.* London, UK: Government of the United Kingdom.

Petasnick, W. D. (2011). End-of-life care: The time for a meaningful discussion is now. *Journal of Healthcare Management, 56,* 369–373.

Phillips, J. L., Halcomb, E. J., & Davidson, P. M. (2011). End-of-life care pathways in acute and hospice care: An integrative review. *Journal of Pain and Symptom Management, 41,* 940–955.

Spinello, I. M. (2011). End-of-life care in ICU: A practical guide. *Journal of Intensive Care Medicine, 26,* 295–303.

Webster, C. R. (2011). End-of-life care pathways for improving outcomes in caring for the dying (review). *The Cochrane Collaboration, 3,* 1–16.

Index